A RIGHT RESULT?

Advocacy, justice and empowerment

Rick Henderson and Mike Pochin

The POLICY

P~P

PRESS

First published in Great Britain in September 2001 by

The Policy Press
University of Bristol
34 Tyndall's Park Road
Bristol BS8 1PY
UK

Tel +44 (0)117 954 6800
Fax +44 (0)117 973 7308
E-mail tpp@bristol.ac.uk
www.policypress.org.uk

ISBN 1 86134 306 X

Rick Henderson is Project Director of Advocacy Across London and
Mike Pochin is a coordinator of Dorset Advocacy.

Cover design by Qube Design Associates, Bristol.

Cover photograph kindly supplied by Ukamaka Bogunjoko.

Printed in Great Britain by Hobbs the Printers Ltd, Southampton.

Contents

Acknowledgements

The authors would like to thank the following for their contributions to the writing of this book:

Hugh Farrell
Robert Weetman
Steve Turner
Sylvia Ellarby
Sally Carr
Joan Taylor
Tricia Banks
Terry and Anne Whitfield
Kathy West
Ukamaka and Tokunbo Bogunjoko
Dorset Health Authority
Advocacy 2000
Drumchapel Advocacy Project
The Advocacy Project (Glasgow)
Merchiston Advocacy Project
Independent Advocacy Service (Southwark)
Southwark Community Care Forum
Advocacy Service Action Project (ASAP)
Choices Advocacy

In addition, we would like to thank all at Dorset Advocacy, and our long-suffering families.

Preface

Books on advocacy, as opposed to self-advocacy, are relatively uncommon. This is surprising given the range and number of advocacy schemes operating within the United Kingdom, all of which reflect in one way or another the core belief that advocacy plays an essential part in securing the rights and protecting the interests of the individual. It is surprising, too, given that advocacy is generally acknowledged to play an important, perhaps a crucial role in the implementation of community care. The concept of advocacy is prominent in local community care plans and charters and in long-stay hospital closure plans. Even central government, which has toyed uneasily with advocacy since the stalling of the 1986 Disabled Persons Act, has now apparently signed up to the idea; advocacy, in the form of Patient Advocacy and Liaison Services (PALS) is to be the lynchpin of this government's National Health Service (NHS) reforms in England and Wales. More recently still, the publication of *Valuing people: A new strategy for learning disability for the 21st century* (DoH, 2001) promises national government funding for the development of advocacy schemes. With mental health reforms in England and Scotland also likely to accord a central role to advocacy, its significance is no longer in doubt.

Why then is there so little literature on advocacy? Two possible reasons have to do with the priorities of advocacy schemes themselves. Citizen advocacy, which was probably the first model of advocacy to become established in the UK, has an inherent suspicion of academic research. It is felt that to research advocacy is to treat it as an 'intervention' and to 'clientise' those it supports, thereby thwarting a key aim of citizen advocacy, which is to promote partners' access to, and acceptance within, the life of the community. Second, the stress laid upon confidentiality by all models of advocacy has led to an understandable reluctance to discuss actual advocacy processes in the public arena.

A third reason may lie in the great diversity of advocacy models now existing within the UK. Professional casework advocacy, citizen advocacy, peer advocacy and volunteer advocacy each have their committed followers who will tend to view their form of advocacy as 'the best'; the debate is only sharpened by the need to compete for scarce funding. The substantial differences between, say, a citizen advocacy scheme that develops advocacy through long-term voluntary partnerships and a scheme that offers short episodes of representation by a trained, paid worker have led people to wonder whether 'advocacy' is really a single concept at all, or simply a name which happens to have been given to a series of more or less separate activities. What is, or is not, true advocacy?

To attempt to write a book about advocacy is to encounter all of these problems, and others besides. We believe the attempt is worthwhile, for several reasons.

First and most simply, advocacy is a force for good, and deserves to be celebrated. This book has been inspired by contact with users of advocacy and with advocacy schemes over a number of years. It is written in the belief that advocacy can bring about significant change not only in the lives of those it supports, but also in social awareness.

Second, advocacy in the UK is facing a series of threats and dilemmas. In part, these reflect the difficulties which invariably beset voluntary sector activities, especially with regard to funding. But the problems also go deeper. As advocacy moves up the political agenda so questions about the nature and quality of advocacy processes are thrown into sharp relief. What *sort* of advocacy should people be entitled to? What distinguishes good advocacy from bad? Unless the advocacy movement can answer these questions, there is a danger that with funding and recognition there may come the imposition of inappropriate standards. Indeed, the proof of Best Value required by local statutory funders of advocacy already threatens to undermine some of its core principles, and to merge its identity with that of wider service provision. Taken together with the recent announcement that Community Health Councils are to be replaced with PALS among other measures (in England at least), it is possible to predict troubled times for the advocacy movement. This book describes many of these challenges and draws out their implications.

It will be suggested that the best way for the 'independent' advocacy movement to counter such difficulties is to demonstrate the integrity and effectiveness of advocacy on its own terms. A third aim of the book, therefore, is to explore the ideas that lie at the heart of advocacy. What sort of perceptions lie behind the different forms of advocacy, and what sort of benefits do they bring about? By clarifying what advocacy is for, it may be possible to lay the foundations for what Dorothy Atkinson calls an autonomous 'advocacy culture' (Atkinson,

1999, p 25). Although the features of such a culture are far from being universally understood or even particularly well defined, there is a real desire within the advocacy movement for a sense of unity, collaboration and coherence. Such a network of ideas and practices may help to prevent advocacy from being diluted or undermined.

Finally, the book aims to explore whether a form of national standards could have a role to play in the development of this advocacy culture, and the ways in which advocacy practice may be strengthened by training and other forms of support for advocates.

Both authors of this book work for advocacy organisations and have (hopefully) absorbed a range of perspectives on advocacy over the years. These work commitments mean that it has not been possible to undertake extensive fieldwork or widespread consultation during the preparation of this book. The present work is above all a book of ideas. Indeed, one of its key themes is the extent to which advocacy is driven by deeply held values and principles. Making sense of advocacy means gaining a clearer picture of these ideas. It is hoped that the book's conclusions will help to carry forward the debates about funding, evaluation and standards in advocacy; but even more importantly that it will help whoever has an interest in advocacy – service users, advocates, funders or policy makers – to reflect on advocacy in their locality, and to contribute to its development.

This is not a book about self-advocacy. It seeks to describe what happens when one person speaks up for, or identifies with, another. However, it may well be that some of the themes presented in this book are familiar to self-advocates; in particular, it is hoped that the outlines of an 'advocacy culture' set out in Chapter Five will be recognisable and useful to them.

Except where indicated otherwise, the stories used to illustrate ideas in the text are invented; that is, they draw on a range of situations which the authors have witnessed or have heard told, but they are not intended to be the stories of real people. In part, this approach reflects the lack of time available for collecting true stories; but it also reflects the concerns for confidentiality stated above. Readers wishing to study accounts of real advocacy partnerships are referred to the inspirational text *Standing by me* (Williams, 1998).

Throughout this work, reference is made to 'care services', 'service workers' and the 'service culture'. A major theme of the book is the way in which the interests of care services may conflict with those of their users. It is also suggested that there are significant tensions between the service culture as represented by the Best Value initiative, and genuinely independent advocacy. None of this should be taken as implying a pejorative view of community care or health services as such. The authors are aware of many services that are genuine and consistent in their commitment to user empowerment; and of many service workers who show tirelessness and skill in pursuit of their clients' interests. It is just as important that advocacy reinforces the efforts of these services and workers as that it challenges poor structures and practices.

A word should be said regarding some of the terms used in this book. For the sake of clarity and consistency, a single set of terms has been used, even though these terms are by no means agreed across the advocacy movement. Advocacy organisations are throughout referred to as 'schemes' rather than 'services', for reasons which should become apparent as the reader progresses. People who are supported by advocates are generally termed 'partners' rather than 'users' or 'clients'. The term 'partner' is widely used in citizen advocacy schemes, but much less so in professional advocacy circles where the whole concept of partnership may seem inapplicable. There were no strong grounds for using 'partner' as opposed to the other terms; we chose it simply because it is unique to the advocacy movement, whereas 'client' and 'user' have wider usage. Different kinds of advocacy (such as volunteer advocacy, professional advocacy) are referred to as 'forms'.

ONE

What is advocacy?

There may be times in all our lives when, for whatever reason, we feel unable to assert ourselves in a given situation. For example, if a waiter in a restaurant delivers the wrong meal or the food arrives lukewarm, we may be reluctant to complain for fear of causing a fuss, and instead allow our (less reticent) dining companion to do so on our behalf. Is this advocacy? If it is, then it can be argued that we can all benefit from advocacy support and can all *be* advocates for those close to us, given the right set of circumstances.

We can all put up with cold food from time to time, but what if the problem is more serious? Suppose a loved one is critically ill in hospital, and it has been suggested that their life-support machine be switched off? The patient cannot make their wishes known, at a time when their vital interests are threatened. The doctors involved will claim to have the patient's best interests at heart, but what if there are another three patients with a 'better' chance of recovery waiting for the intensive care bed? In wanting the best for these patients also, the doctors have a conflict of interests. All sorts of questions might go through our minds in this situation. Do the doctors realise how precious this person is? Have they really done all that can be done? Are they sure of their diagnosis? We might articulate some or all of these questions, prompted by a sense that the patient deserves no less. In doing so, we are acting as their advocate.

Advocacy can be described as the process of identifying with and representing a person's views and concerns, in order to secure enhanced rights and entitlements, undertaken by someone who has little or no conflict of interest. Put more positively, advocacy is rooted in a special, and perhaps unique, relationship between the advocate and the person they support and uses the tools of representation, negotiation and persuasion in order to bring about a beneficial change in the partner's life. Advocacy requires a commitment to the 'partner' (the term that will be used throughout this book for the person supported by an advocate) but also a determination to see the process through – to aim for something better at the end of the process, either a concrete 'victory' (such as a change of residential home or a new social worker), or a greater sense of involvement and empowerment. This book aims to reflect on the processes and presuppositions that are involved when one person speaks up for another, and the ways in which advocacy organisations in the UK have codified these processes. It will reflect on the main strengths and weaknesses of advocacy, and suggest ways in which the advocacy movement could develop.

The need for advocacy arises where circumstances have taken away an individual's ability to speak up freely for their interests. The advocacy movement has at its foundations the recognition that there are groups of people for whom such radical disempowerment is not so much a random occurrence as a way of life. This book will study the particular forms of advocacy which have at their core the active representation of the views and interests of people who are at significant risk of social exclusion or misrepresentation. The main forms of advocacy can be introduced as follows.

Citizen advocacy

The real roots of contemporary advocacy can be traced to the United States and attempts to address the fears and anxieties of carers and families of disabled people. The opening statement of the seminal British text *Citizen advocacy: A powerful partnership* (Butler et al, 1988) accurately summarises the birth of the citizen advocacy movement:

> ... in 1966, delegates at a conference in the United States, concerned with cerebral palsy, looked at the question 'What will happen to my child when I'm gone?' They decided that one answer might be that when there is no family, willing or able, to protect a person's interests, those interests could continue to be protected by a 'citizen advocate', an unpaid citizen who has no connection with the service provided to that person, thus avoiding any conflict of interest. (Butler et al, 1988, p 3)

With the identification of vulnerable groups and of social and service structures whose interests may always conflict with those of the individual, came the inspiration for organised advocacy. The concept was seized upon and developed by people concerned with issues of rights and protection for vulnerable people, notably Wolf

Wolfensberger (and his collaborators) and John O'Brien. Wolfensberger in particular can be credited with defining and promoting a set of guiding principles for the emerging citizen advocacy movement that continue to predominate. His model was based on a long-term, one-to-one relationship between the advocate (who should be an independent, unpaid and valued member of the local community) and their partner or 'protégé'. The primary role of the citizen advocate was to promote and where necessary represent, the interests and wishes of their partner. Although citizen advocates would be recruited, 'matched' and supported by their local scheme, their primary loyalty would be to their partner.

Citizen advocacy philosophy can be seen to be guided by a number of assumptions about society and about those service systems that are designed to care for and support vulnerable people. The first of these is that certain groups of people are at great risk of exclusion and ill-treatment, not only from society at large, but also from the very service systems which are designed to care for them. These groups could include (but are not limited to) older people; people with mental health problems; people with learning disabilities; people with physical and sensory disabilities; people living with HIV and AIDS; homeless people; people with drug or alcohol problems; and children with special needs or 'looked after'. To a large extent, the history of care for such groups of people is a history of institutionalisation, abuse and neglect. While there has been a great deal of progress in relation to the shift away from large, Victorian hospitals towards community-based alternatives, these new services, although *based* in the community, are often not *part* of the community. To this extent Wolfensberger's perceptions of exclusion and potential abuse still seem valid. There are many instances where current statutory powers have proved inadequate to protect service users. Where such powers do exist, the interests of the public (for example, the drive to maintain low income tax rates) may not coincide with the interests of those who require state support as a result of age, disability or poverty.

The second key assumption is that there are people who care enough about the situation described above to voluntarily give up their time to do something about it. In essence, this is what makes citizen advocacy unique and is one of its key selling points. Wolfensberger's assertion was that ordinary US citizens could and should give a commitment to engaging in mutually beneficial relationships with people who were at risk of social exclusion or worse, in a spirit of community integration. To the extent that citizen advocacy schemes based on Wolfensberger's vision have proliferated both in the US and across the globe, then he could be said to have guessed right. However, the concept of the 'valued citizen' as a central tenet of citizen advocacy philosophy remains as contentious now as it ever was three decades ago. Essentially, the debate hinges on whether it is possible to define a person's 'value' as a constant, unchanging attribute or whether it is in fact, specific only to particular situations and environments. Features such as race, gender, religion and social class can all have a bearing on an individual's standing and credibility, but they do not in themselves define value or status. Many of Wolfensberger's critics have argued that his benchmark for the valued citizen is the white, middle-class male (see, for example, Chappell, 1992). Although Wolfensberger himself has vigorously denied this, the legacy of such an indictment lives on. Many contemporary UK citizen advocacy schemes have substituted the phrase 'valued citizen' with the less contentious 'ordinary person' in order to counter the supposition that some citizens are inherently more suitable to become advocates than others.

Citizen advocacy: key features

Advocates are unpaid members of the local community

Long-term, one-to-one relationship

Schemes actively seek out individuals who may benefit from a citizen advocacy relationship

Advocacy scheme 'matches' advocate and partner

Advocate is accountable principally to their partner

Schemes are structurally independent from service agencies

Citizen advocacy continues to be influential in the UK, with dozens of schemes subscribing to many if not all of the principles outlined by Wolfensberger. Although there are citizen advocacy schemes supporting older people and those with mental health problems, the largest number of schemes create partnerships with people who have learning disabilities. The long-term nature of citizen advocacy partnerships offers the potential for developing self-confidence and opportunities with those who may have experienced exclusion and institutionalisation over many years. In particular, citizen advocacy more than any other advocacy form allows for the active identification of those individuals who may benefit from an advocacy relationship even if they are not able to refer themselves to a scheme. Citizen advocacy principles assert that many people who might gain most from such a partnership are those who are least likely to put themselves forward (the 'least vocal, least visible, most vulnerable' members of society). Some citizen advocacy schemes adopt a policy of 'assertive outreach' within service systems, paying regular visits to settings such as day centres, residential homes and hospital wards to identify potential partners and make them aware of the scheme. At best, such an assertive approach represents a significant step towards the social inclusion of the most isolated members of the community. However, this needs to be tempered with a respect for privacy and confidentiality and an understanding that some individuals will choose not to engage with citizen advocacy schemes or advocates at all.

Citizen advocacy principles allow for the recruitment of a small number of short-term or crisis advocates within schemes. Such advocates help individuals to resolve a given problem, and then withdraw, rather than offering the ongoing support typical of citizen advocacy. Given the difficulties which many people experience in accessing community care and other entitlements, it is not surprising that this form of advocacy has taken on a life of its own. Throughout the book, we have referred to it as volunteer advocacy.

Volunteer advocacy

Volunteer advocacy schemes share with their citizen advocacy counterparts the belief that the unpaid status of the advocate is of primary importance. Advocates speak up for their partners out of commitment to them, and not for remuneration. However, such schemes are likely to take a pragmatic approach to the paying of volunteer expenses, whereas most citizen advocacy schemes would view even this as diluting the advocate's loyalty to the partner.

Volunteer advocacy schemes are more likely to be 'generic' than citizen advocacy ones; that is, they will work with a range of partners who may be disabled, elderly, or mental health users, or who may not identify with any particular group. Because the advocacy is issues-based, the advocates support a number of advocacy partners. Whereas the 'match' between advocate and partner is likely to be the determining factor in the success or failure of a citizen advocacy partnership, volunteer advocacy will depend as much on the knowledge and skill of the advocate as on their relationship with the partner. Training and supervision of advocates are therefore likely to be prominent features of volunteer advocacy schemes.

Volunteer advocacy: key features
Advocates give their time freely although they may receive out-of-pocket expenses
Partnerships focus on resolving specific issues rather than on long-term support
Advocates may support more than one partner at a time
Schemes are likely to support a range of user groups

Self-advocacy

The growth of citizen advocacy and other forms of 'third-party' advocacy schemes has coincided with the development of a burgeoning self-advocacy movement and the establishment of user-led organisations such as Survivors Speak Out (mental health user network) and People First (self-advocacy groups of people with learning disabilities). There are now a large number of local, regional and national user organisations which share the common objectives of empowerment, pride and social justice. Most of these are organised around a specific issue or client group although some are broad-based coalitions of groups and individuals. Although such groups may have shared aims and aspirations, they differ widely in their choice of methods by which to achieve them. These range from information and mutual support to political lobbying and direct action. User groups may also engage in awareness-raising and training activities as well as supporting group members to learn new skills and develop self-confidence.

Self-advocacy has been perhaps the predominant form of advocacy adopted by (physically) disabled people. Local coalitions of disabled people, often affiliated to the British Council of Organisations of Disabled People (BCODP), have vigorously asserted their members' equality and right to independence. These groups have at times voiced criticism of citizen and other forms of advocacy on the grounds that they may perpetuate perceptions of the essential dependency of disabled people.

Self-advocacy: key features

Organised and driven by disabled people or service users

Self-advocacy groups offer mutual support and confidence building

Individuals working together to challenge stereotypes and discrimination

Operating at local and national level

Sharing information, knowledge and experience

Peer advocacy

The term 'peer advocacy' is used to describe advocacy relationships in which both the advocate and their partner share a common experience or environment, for example, two residents in a nursing home, two patients in a general practice, or two women with personal experience of domestic violence. Although peer advocacy is not in itself a discrete advocacy form in the same way as, say, citizen advocacy, it can nevertheless provide a powerful force for both challenge and change within service settings. Peer advocacy refers primarily to *who* does the advocacy, rather than *how* it is done. Peer advocates (whose primary qualification is their own personal experience of disability, service usage or dis/empowerment) may engage in a one-to-one relationship; have a caseload of clients; or support a self-advocacy group. There are a small number of specific peer advocacy schemes in the UK (for example the Peer Advocacy Project at the Maudsley Hospital, London) but the model of advocacy practised by such schemes is not clearly defined. Often, peer advocacy occurs in an informal and often impromptu way within service settings such as day centres, residential homes and hospital wards.

Ethel

Ethel is waiting to see her GP. As she sits in the waiting room, she notices that the elderly woman sitting beside her is becoming more and more distressed. Ethel decides to intervene:

"Are you alright, dear?"

"Not really, I've been waiting for ages and I'm not feeling too good."

"How long have you been waiting exactly?"

"Two hours. I think they've forgotten about me but I don't want to make a fuss."

"Two hours? That's outrageous! Why don't you let me have a word with the receptionist, just to check how much longer you have to wait? It's no trouble."

Ethel speaks to the receptionist on her peer's behalf and argues for her to be given priority in the queue.

As well as being a genuine act of human kindness and solidarity, the actions of Ethel in the vignette above are also inherently *political*, in that they provide a challenge to widely-held beliefs that only those with high status within society are able to effect change. At one level, Ethel is as disempowered as her frustrated peer – she too is elderly, a patient, stuck in an inhospitable doctor's waiting room – but for whatever reason, she feels both willing and able to intervene. Given another set of circumstances, it may be Ethel herself who benefits from her peer's intervention, and in time both parties may come to enjoy a fruitful and mutually beneficial relationship.

Peer advocacy: key features

Advocate and partner share common experiences or environments

Relationship often based on mutual support and empowerment

Peer advocacy may be one-to-one or casework-based

Few established peer advocacy schemes

Peer advocates challenge power dynamics of 'giver' and 'receiver'

Professional casework advocacy

In the field of mental health, especially within the psychiatric hospital system with its emphasis on compulsion and detention, an alternative form of advocacy was found in the Dutch patients' advocate approach. This introduced the concept of the advocate as paid worker, with a 'caseload' of clients who sought support with a range of issues (see, for example, Klijnsma, 1993). In recent years this form has been imported into the community, and not only in a mental health context – the most rapid growth in advocacy has been in such professional casework schemes covering a wide range of client groups. There may be a number of reasons for this, including: the general decline in the number of volunteers coupled with an increase in the range of voluntary work opportunities; the crisis nature of many people's problems; and the potential for a professional casework advocacy scheme to support larger numbers of people than its citizen advocacy counterpart. This latter point may make such a scheme more attractive to funding bodies who feel it will give them 'more' advocacy for their money. Statutory funding agencies may also believe that a professional casework scheme can be more accountable or even more 'professional' in its approach although there is little empirical evidence to support this claim. However, such a close alliance with the statutory sector certainly increases the potential for a conflict of interest to arise. Although paid advocates may have a better knowledge of local services and systems (as they are working within them on a daily basis) there is a greater danger of collusion with service agencies and the threat of withdrawal of funding if the advocate behaves in ways which offend the statutory services.

It is within professional casework advocacy schemes that the impetus for more consistent standards, accreditation and regulation is most strongly felt and articulated. To the extent that relatively high levels of public resources are being targeted towards this type of advocacy, such a focus may be appropriate, but there is a danger that the drive for greater accountability will lead to the imposition of traditional service measures which value quantity over quality. At its best, professional casework advocacy combines a values-driven focus on relationships, empathy and solidarity with a high level of expertise in and knowledge of local service systems and how to effect change on behalf of individuals within those systems. Although casework advocacy does not have the same emphasis on long-term, one-to-one relationships as citizen advocacy, it does have a crucial role to play in ensuring that people's rights and entitlements are safeguarded on a day-to-day basis.

Professional casework advocacy: key features
Advocates are generally paid workers
Each advocate has a 'caseload' of people they support
Advocacy is task-based, with clear outcomes and targets
Advocate/partner relationships are usually short-term in nature
Advocates work in a team

Legal advocacy

Legal advocacy is best seen as a separate but complementary form of advocacy to those described elsewhere in this chapter. In this context the term 'legal advocacy' is used to refer to the work done by lawyers on behalf of users of health and social care services (in the form of litigation and judicial reviews) and those investigations carried out by quasi-legal bodies such as ombudsmen. The relevance for this chapter is that advocacy schemes often refer complex cases or those where there is believed to be a legal precedent, to law centres, legal practices or, in the case of complaints, to the relevant ombudsman (there are ombudsmen for the NHS, local authorities and the independent housing sector).

In a legal context, advocacy can be seen to mean 'representing' or 'pleading a case on behalf of' an individual. In order for this representation to be effective, there needs to be some degree of legal precedent, that is, an existing law applies or a new law needs to be made on the strength of a particular case. Examples of this include challenging a local authority's duty of care, contesting the imposition of a Mental Health Act section or suing for medical negligence. But the term advocacy is used to describe the particular activity of lawyers and other legal professionals rather than in the 'cultural' context applied elsewhere in this book. Legal advocacy is different to other advocacy forms in a number of very important respects.

It is common for advocacy schemes to develop relationships with lawyers or law practices specialising in particular issues such as mental health or housing. Many schemes have lawyers on the management committee as a means of obtaining legal expertise within the scheme. Conversely, many solicitors' firms have close links with local 'lay' advocacy schemes and refer on to them if a case is unlikely to be successful in a court of law. This is especially relevant in the context of community care where so much of what happens is governed not by laws, but by local policies and procedures. However, Bateman (2000) insists that:

> While some advocacy can be performed successfully using good negotiation skills, without relying on the law or other rules, it is not advisable, and it is important to establish whether there is a legal basis to a case before commencing negotiations or any other active advocacy. (Bateman, 2000, p 138)

This may well be overstating the case for legal intervention. Lay advocates (a legal term to describe non-legal advocacy) have the added advantage of being better able to develop longer-term relationships with partners that are not exclusively outcome-focused and may ultimately prove more rewarding to both advocate and partner. There is also the issue of cost – taking a case through the courts can be an extremely expensive business, and changes to legal aid structures have made it much more difficult for individuals to obtain financial assistance in fighting their case. Even Bateman himself goes on to state that people often

> ... require skilled, appropriate legal help. Despite this, there are many instances where the client does not have access to skilled, appropriate legal help. (Bateman, 2000, p 138)

Brandon (1995) is more critical of the legal profession, especially in relation to people with disabilities. He suggests that, through lawyers' self-appointed 'expert' status and desire for profit, they reproduce many of the power imbalances that already exist in the wider society. He goes on to argue that:

> The movement from domination by care professionals to domination by lawyers can consist in simply swapping one form of tyranny for another. (Brandon, 1995, p 18)

According to Bateman (2000, ch 11) there are six stages to advocacy in a legal context: presentation; information–gathering; legal research; interpretation and feedback; active negotiation and advocacy; and litigation. It is telling to note that at no point during this process is the advocate required to develop anything other than a cursory relationship with their 'client' – they are entirely focused on obtaining an outcome based on the facts of the case. In this way, it is unlikely that the person on the receiving end of the legal advocate's intervention will have any opportunity to represent themselves (self-advocacy), learn new skills or even gain new experience.

Legal advocacy: key features	
Legal advocacy	**'Lay' advocacy**
Professional service model	Variety of advocacy forms
Lawyers as 'experts'	Advocates as 'knowledgeable allies'
Based on legal precedence	Based on rights, choice and justice
Outcome-focused	Process- *and* outcome-focused
Service often fee-based	Free to partners

What has advocacy achieved in the UK?

Spend a day with almost any established advocacy scheme in the UK and you are likely to come away with a sense of something new and exciting going on. Whatever hard evidence there may or may not be for outcomes (and of this more later) the advocacy movement as a whole sustains levels of enthusiasm and commitment found in few other fields of social endeavour. Hearing anecdotes from schemes, one is struck again and again by the twin themes of the recovery of human dignity and the lifting of 'social censorship' – challenging those attitudes and structures which impose a kind of silence on the individual. Twenty years into the history of the UK advocacy movement, these themes show no sign of exhaustion; on the contrary, they seem to reflect and may even have shaped (if the main political parties are to be believed) a political culture which aspires to the dismantling of all barriers to individual opportunity.

Nor is this sense of conviction limited to the advocacy movement itself. Advocacy enjoys generally high repute among social services and NHS providers. Advocacy has both shaped and benefited from the culture of care in the community, which at least purports to promote choice and user-centredness. The restrictive professional practices of the hospital era, by which medical staff could define a patient's interests without fear of challenge, have waned considerably. The right to advocacy is stated in many local Community Care Charters (although perhaps without guarantee that a local scheme exists to provide it) and good practice guidelines at both national and local level extol the virtue of an advocate's involvement. When service workers *are* critical of advocacy, it is generally of a particular scheme's failure to live up to its ideals – not of the ideal itself.

With dynamism and respect has come growth. In 20 years, literally hundreds of schemes have developed across the UK. There has been continued innovation and adaptation: the citizen advocacy form has been successfully applied in both urban and rural settings, and has supported people of all ages and from a range of minority ethnic groups. Equally, alternative models such as self, peer or casework advocacy have evolved according to local needs and ideas. In particular, these last-named models of advocacy have been taken up as part of wider actions for social change. Many social campaign groups now include individual advocacy among their programmes of action.

What has the UK advocacy movement failed to achieve?

We have so far spoken of the 'advocacy movement' as though the existence of this were an established fact. On closer inspection, this turns out to be far from certain. Ask the question 'What is advocacy?' of five advocacy schemes, and their five answers may have little in common. For a start, there are very diverse forms of advocacy each operating to principles that are not only different, but may appear contradictory. For example, citizen advocacy schemes champion the idea of the untrained advocate, the ordinary citizen who is uncontaminated by service perspectives; casework advocate schemes will tend to emphasise the importance of knowing 'the system' well, so as to champion the user whose rights are threatened by it. Some groups will see advocacy as an activity which must be kept distinct, whereas for others it may be part of a wider movement for social change, blending with other features such as advice, information-giving or befriending. Even among advocacy groups of the same type, there may be strong disagreements about, for example, the precise extent of users' confidentiality, or whether or not volunteer advocates should receive expenses.

So, for all the movement's dynamism, advocacy lacks a clear *identity*. This is reflected in the fact that while service providers in many instances accord advocacy a high status, it is barely recognised, let alone understood by most members of the public. The term 'advocacy' itself sounds awkward and specialist – no great help if one is really trying to convey the message that most members of the community may both *need advocacy* and *be advocates* themselves at one time or another in their lives.

Not surprisingly, this lack of identity has undermined most attempts to formulate and develop good practice across advocacy schemes. The organisation Citizen Advocacy Information and Training (CAIT) has long been the national resource for citizen advocacy schemes. Over the past 15 years, it has promoted a set of principles and a Code of Practice which define citizen advocacy, and has supported coordinators' forums at which practice issues can be shared. Much good work has been done here, but it is a fact that a significant (and perhaps growing) number of schemes do not wish to follow the citizen advocacy model. Similarly, the United Kingdom Advocacy Network (UKAN) has done substantial work with mental health user groups, and has also produced a Code of Practice for advocates (UKAN, 1997); but this too is specific to one form of advocacy. Thus at the regional level, one finds a series of forums (for example Advocacy Across London, Wessex Advocacy Consortium) which represent the many different kinds of schemes. However, what these bodies gain in inclusivity, they tend to lose in political force; they are unable to lay down local standards for advocacy, or to issue authoritative guidelines to purchasers, precisely because they embody such diversity.

There is, then, a lack of *coherence* in the advocacy movement; on the one hand no national body commands the widespread assent required for its code and principles to become standard; on the other, regional forums lack the unanimity to develop such standards for their own members. Whether the new National Citizen Advocacy Network envisaged by the government (DoH, 2001) can resolve this paradox remains to be seen.

With this lack of coherence comes a still more worrying lack of *consistency*. If advocacy is known for its dynamism and strong values base, it also has a reputation for variability in its success rate:

"In another instance, his advocate was having such a detrimental effect on Bob that Bob's brother asked that the advocate be removed. The care manager had to become involved and scrutinise the quality of the advocacy service being provided. Subsequently the advocacy group apologised for the advocate, and he was withdrawn." (Christina Wiggin, presentation to BILD Citizen Advocacy Conference, London, March 2000)

In this instance, something clearly was wrong with the advocate; but there have been many other instances where family members have 'asked that the advocate be removed' for all the wrong reasons. For example, the advocate may be trying to help the partner to assert their right to control their own finances in the face of opposition from family members who are either over-protective or (sadly, as sometimes happens) using the money for their own purposes. What criteria exist to distinguish 'good' from 'bad' advocacy, and who applies them? Though social services seem to have assumed this 'judicial' role in the anecdote about Bob, above, they can hardly be allowed to sit in permanent judgement of schemes that are, often, challenging them.

There are a couple of models of evaluation current within the citizen advocacy movement, but these have no formal status; at best, they constitute a form of peer review. For the wider advocacy movement, there seem to be no agreed benchmarks for performance whatsoever. This has in recent years led to a tendency for purchasers of advocacy (primarily health and social services) to impose their own monitoring regimes on local advocacy schemes. We shall argue that this threatens to turn advocacy into a 'numbers game', while yielding little useful information about its value and favouring quantitative rather than qualitative outcome measures.

Government initiatives will undoubtedly develop the statutory basis of advocacy over the next few years. But what sort of advocacy will this be? The various forms of advocacy described in this chapter are all dynamic and influential; but they are also typically delivered by schemes which are informal, diverse, and locally-based. Is there a danger that with statutory recognition there may come a demand for the standardisation of advocacy which will threaten its key principles and vitality? The authors of this work believe that just such a threat does exist, but that it can be averted by clear thinking and common action on the part of advocacy organisations.

Advocacy is an act of solidarity between two people. It is a political act with consequences for both individuals and the community as a whole, challenging inequality, opposing racism, preventing abuse, or even introducing someone to a new opportunity or social setting – all constituting steps towards a more civil and just society. But planning, implementing and supporting advocacy is not straightforward. The next chapter will highlight some of the difficulties that beset advocacy schemes.

TWO

Issues in contemporary advocacy

In Chapter One we described the history and development of the UK advocacy movement, from its origins in the US citizen advocacy doctrine through to contemporary forms of casework, peer and generic advocacy provision. This rapid expansion in the number and type of local schemes has undoubtedly meant that many more people have benefited from advocacy support than would otherwise have done so. Within the context of diminishing resources and increased need for primary health and social care services, this can only be a good thing. Advocacy plays a key role in ensuring that people's voices are heard, their views heeded and acted on. It can be argued that as a direct result of the intervention of advocates, a great many more people have access to the types of care and support they need to live full and active lives. Advocates have secured extra resources, battled against institutionalisation, challenged bad practice and pioneered acceptance and tolerance. Above all, advocates have championed the cause of the individual within a system that seems to be predisposed towards categorisation and depersonalisation.

Although there is much to justify the celebration of these achievements, there remain a number of fundamental dilemmas for the advocacy movement that, if not addressed, may pose a very real threat to its continued progress. In attempting to define these dilemmas, we accept that there will be a range of views about the relative priority of such issues. Nonetheless, we hope that by naming the problems, by stimulating debate both within the movement and with those individuals and agencies affected by advocacy, real solutions can begin to be developed.

Advocacy in the UK has developed rapidly in the last 20 years. It is not surprising that most energy should have been expended on defining the principles which make each form of advocacy distinct, and on building local schemes which enshrine these principles. However, this emphasis on ideology and local action could lead to advocacy becoming essentially inward looking if it is not balanced by broader perspectives. There is a need to identify, develop and share good practice if advocacy is to have a strong national profile. More pressing still, there is a need to recognise the common threats facing advocacy schemes, to understand their implications, and to agree remedies.

Six issues in particular present difficulties for contemporary advocacy:

Problems for UK advocacy schemes

The need for secure *funding*

Maintaining real *independence* in advocacy

Ensuring *equity* and a diverse spectrum of advocacy arrangements for a multicultural society

Defining and promoting *loyalty* to the partner

Minimising *risk* to both advocates and partners

Demonstrating effectiveness and accountability (via *regulation, evaluation and training*) without compromising principles

Each of these issues deserves to be examined in greater detail.

Funding

It is fair to say that the majority of advocacy schemes in this country are still dependent on the statutory sector funding available primarily via health authorities and social services departments. Although this financial support is welcome and serves to provide stability and security to local advocacy projects, there are inherent dangers in relying too heavily on such funding. Primarily, these centre on the potential for a conflict of interest to arise when advocacy services attempt to assert their independence on behalf of local service users. Advocates often find themselves in the unenviable position of 'biting the hand that feeds them', for example when advocating for users whose services have been cut or reduced by the funding authority. There is also a danger of losing credibility with potential users of the advocacy scheme as a result of not being truly independent. How can users trust the scheme's promise of confidentiality and loyalty if it is funded by the very bodies that have failed them? It is incumbent on advocacy projects to develop positive strategies for combating these dilemmas, such as the negotiation of contracts that ensure autonomy can be safeguarded even when relations between the two parties become strained. It is perfectly feasible that such schemes can be funded on the explicit understanding that the advocacy role can be adversarial even though partnership working is preferential. In many areas codes of practice have been jointly developed between funding bodies and advocacy schemes which detail how advocacy support is to be provided, to which client groups and by which methods. The following is an extract from a 'Statement of operational principles' developed by Advocacy Partners:

> An advocate as a free and independent agent shall determine his/her own actions in relation to the needs of his/her partner. Neither a service agency nor the Citizen Advocacy office can order an advocate how to act on behalf of the partner whom he/she represents. (quoted in Wertheimer, 1998, p 90)

While advocacy codes of practice can offer some safeguards against bad practice and serve to clarify the respective duties of both parties, it is essential that they are not dictatorial to the extent of stifling creativity. The desired outcomes, and the processes adopted to achieve them, should remain within the control of the advocate/partner relationship.

In recent years many large regional and national charities have set their sights on advocacy provision. For these organisations, advocacy is only one small aspect of a much larger portfolio which may include direct service provision. In many areas, such 'corporate' schemes are now in the majority, especially where the funding agencies have insisted on a competitive tendering process that favours those organisations familiar with such business practices. Few local schemes have the infrastructure necessary to compete in such an arena, even though they may have the advantages of local knowledge and support from local users and service agencies. Nor is competitive tendering the only way in which the contract culture has affected advocacy provision. Statutory funders increasingly demand evidence of value for money or 'Best Value'. This raises again the question 'what is good advocacy?'

Ironically, the advocacy scheme may also find itself *competing* with service provider agencies for scarce resources at a local level. The proportion of those resources that are allocated to each activity will probably depend as much on politics as it does on need. For funding bodies, especially the key agencies of health and social services, the decision to fund advocacy is driven by a reluctant acknowledgement of the existence of deficiencies in service provision. Put another way, advocacy services exist and are funded to *point out the gaps* in services, in order that commissioners and service planners may address them. In a system as complex and multifaceted as community care, there will always be people who slip through the net. Experience shows that more often than not, the victims of this anomaly are those individuals and groups of people who are similarly disadvantaged in other arenas of public life: women, black and minority ethnic communities, gay men and lesbians. Even within service systems devised specifically to support frail and vulnerable people, such inequalities can be found in both the commissioning and provision of care. By targeting resources towards advocacy, statutory agencies are opening themselves up to challenge and scrutiny of both their philosophy and practice (although the extent to which this is legislation driven rather than undertaken voluntarily is open to question). Advocates for disadvantaged people will eagerly take issue with service providers on their clients' behalf, ensuring users' views and concerns are taken up and acted on by the relevant personnel. In so doing, advocates are operating within a political context, challenging the status quo and providing a force for change; thus there is an inherent potential for conflict between independent advocacy and statutory funders.

Salvation from such dilemmas can come in the form of non-statutory, independent funding such as that available via the many charitable trusts (and, of course, the National Lottery) which provide resources to voluntary organisations. But even these have their own problems such as the short-term nature of funding, usually up to a maximum of three years, and the need to make the project comply with funders' particular criteria. Trusts will not always be fully appraised of the need for advocacy or how best to support its development. When funding does run out, schemes are often faced with the unenviable task of ending advocacy relationships or leaving them unsupported. Although continuation funding can sometimes be forthcoming, many statutory bodies are reluctant to offer resources to schemes previously funded by grant-making trusts and vice versa. Hence, the reality for the majority of advocacy schemes is that long-term funding is far from secure.

Traditional citizen advocacy schemes, following Wolfensberger, have pursued 'multi-source' funding as a solution to this problem. This means having a wide range of funding sources which may include the statutory sector, charitable trusts, private sector sponsorship or assistance in kind, and income generation from activities such as training and consultancy. One downside to such an approach is that the amount of administrative resources needed increases proportionately with the number of contributors. There may be a need for a fundraising post to be created as well as additional bookkeeping and financial control procedures. There may also be different monitoring requirements for each funding body. For example, social services departments may require 'hard' measures such as number of clients seen, length of interventions and so on, whereas charitable donors may be more concerned with quality of life indices. The more an advocacy scheme must 'build capacity' to deal with these demands, the greater the likelihood of tension between bureaucratic structures on the one hand, and user-centredness on the other.

The potential for direct government funding for advocacy is an issue of ongoing debate. The 1986 Disabled Persons (Services, Consultation and Representation) Act first raised the possibility of legislative recognition of the need for independent advocacy and for this to be funded centrally. The original intention was for disabled people to be given the legal right to an advocate when required. Although this key section of the Act was not implemented by the then Conservative government, the campaign for legal recognition of advocacy began in earnest. While the value of advocacy was noted in subsequent legislation, such as the 1990 National Health Service and Community Care Act, state involvement in the funding and development of a comprehensive programme of advocacy provision was not forthcoming. The issue has been raised again in the context of the government review of the 1983 Mental Health Act, with mental health advocacy schemes across the country instrumental in lobbying for access to independent advocates to be made a statutory right.

Most recently, the learning disabilities White Paper *Valuing people: A new strategy for learning disability for the 21st century* (DoH, 2001) has at least conceded the principle of central government funding for advocacy. The White Paper commits the government to the twin aims of setting up a National Citizen Advocacy Network and ensuring that there is resourcing for a citizen advocacy scheme in every local authority area. The medium-term future of advocacy will to a considerable extent hinge on the success or failure of these plans.

In a general health context, the recent announcement in the NHS Plan (DoH, 2000) that the government intends to introduce a network of Patients Advocacy and Liaison Schemes (PALS), has sent shock waves through an understandably cynical advocacy movement. Although the development of PALS will present opportunities for the advocacy movement both in terms of recognition that advocacy is a force for good, and as a possible source of funding, there seems a real danger that PALS will be advocacy in name only. The very fact that advocacy is used in conjunction with the concept of 'liaison' suggests that PALS may be as much about the needs of the system as of individual patients. More will be said of this later.

Independence

Project and advocate independence is crucial for a number of key reasons. Advocacy is about being loyal or 'partial' (as opposed to impartial) to the people advocated for, hence the first line of accountability is justifiably to service users. Often, users come to advocacy schemes as a last resort, after their own efforts to resolve issues and problems have failed – and for many potential users, even approaching the scheme is in itself a huge achievement. Indeed, some advocacy schemes, particularly citizen advocacy schemes, are proactive in offering advocacy to individuals for this very reason; they may lack the confidence to ask for support. It is an indictment of our current system that many individuals will have developed a deep sense of mistrust of conventional services as a result of previous bad experiences. At its most extreme, many within service systems (particularly those who have experienced a lifetime of institutionalisation or 'care') have encountered real abuse and neglect at the hands of those who were supposed to protect them. There is no shortage of examples of vulnerable people being sexually, emotionally, physically and financially abused in service settings such as children's homes, psychiatric hospitals and residential care homes. In order for the advocacy scheme to truly represent these users' views it needs to be free from conflict of interest, able to promise loyalty to users without compromise and strong enough to challenge authority on behalf of individuals.

There are a whole range of ways in which independence impacts on both the design and implementation of advocacy programmes.

These include organisational structure; ownership of the scheme and its work; selection, training and support of advocates.

Organisational structure and ownership

Many advocacy schemes are independently managed, either as registered charities or companies limited by guarantee (or both), with their own, independently elected management committees comprising interested and skilled local people. This is the ideal model as it promotes autonomy and safeguards the schemes' principles from corruption or outside influence. However, it can also be the most difficult to achieve and sustain. Recruiting enthusiastic and committed volunteers to act as trustees for the agency can be extremely difficult, especially given that advocacy must compete with more well-known causes such as care of older people or children's services. Advocacy as a concept is still not well understood by the general public and hence those people who may be interested in joining a management committee may not be aware of the existence of local advocacy schemes or may be hesitant about getting involved in an activity about which they have little knowledge. However, once such schemes are established they are often very popular with users, who perceive them as truly independent and best able to fight their cause without fear of compromise. Involving users in the day-to-day running and management of the scheme may further enhance independence. In this way, users are not just on the receiving end of the advocacy process, they are also directing its implementation.

Not all advocacy schemes enjoy such independence, however. Some other schemes are less structurally independent, being run as projects within larger voluntary organisations such as the National Schizophrenia Fellowship, MENCAP and Age Concern. Others still are managed by local infrastructure organisations such as Councils for Voluntary Service (CVS) until such time as they achieve independence in their own right. In these instances a different kind of independence takes priority. Although not structurally independent in the way described above, it is essential that the schemes aspire towards *operational independence*: in other words, their efforts on behalf of service users are autonomous and unconstrained. However, the relationship between advocacy and wider voluntary sector endeavours may also be fraught with difficulties. As the voluntary sector has embraced contracting and there has been an unprecedented shift towards not only general service provision but more specifically the rebranding and repackaging of traditional statutory services within the voluntary sector, so the advocacy movement has found itself at odds with those who would previously have been allies and colleagues. Consider this example:

Common roots, conflicting interests?

Anytown Older Peoples Project (AOPP) started out as a social club for elderly residents of Anytown, run exclusively by volunteers and supported by the local Council for Voluntary Service (CVS). However, the advent of community care and the contract culture meant that AOPP was suddenly in demand as a provider of day care to a much wider client group, including those with dementia, older people from minority ethnic communities and carers. As a result of a number of astute funding bids, AOPP is now employing 35 staff across five sites, with a further three day centres due to come on stream in the next 18 months. The next priority will be to develop low-cost domiciliary care to older people in their own homes plus a 'put-to-bed' scheme for older people with dementia. In addition, AOPP has recently won the contract to manage the meals-on-wheels scheme previously run by the local council.

Anytown Advocacy Service (AAS) also began life as a volunteer-led project supported by the CVS. Although not exclusively an older peoples' project, AAS is currently funded to provide advocacy to a wide range of local service users in relation to their care and support needs. The project staff and volunteers have become increasingly concerned about the number of complaints they have received about the quality of services offered by AOPP, particularly in relation to staff shortages in the day centres and the poor quality of meals-on-wheels. However, the AAS has come under pressure from other staff within the CVS to 'go easy' on AOPP, especially given their common roots.

It is because of such conflicts of interests that the advocacy sector has fiercely maintained its independence, remaining aloof and somewhat detached from other voluntary sector service providers. Although advocacy is often characterised by its relationship with the statutory agencies of health, housing and social services, it is just as likely that an advocacy scheme will be required to challenge bad practice in a voluntary organisation with charitable aims ostensibly similar to its own.

A central tenet of all forms of advocacy is that the advocate, whether paid worker or volunteer, citizen advocate or caseworker, has the autonomy and strength of character to act independently on behalf of their partner or client. The question for those charged with the responsibility for ensuring this happens (in other words, scheme coordinators and managers) is the extent to which such independence can be achieved within a structure that does not have advocacy as its core purpose.

Selection and support of advocates

It is not enough for advocacy schemes to simply be structurally or operationally independent. The real test of that independence is the extent to which advocates themselves are operating in a client-led, autonomous fashion. This has implications for both the recruitment, training and ongoing support of advocates, whether paid workers or volunteers. An effective advocate may possess (or at least aspire to) any number of useful attributes including tenacity, patience, empathy and optimism. There is also a whole range of appropriate skills that would prove beneficial, such as active listening, letter and report writing, negotiation and communication skills and a working knowledge of relevant legislation. It is up to individual advocacy schemes to decide how these skills and traits will be identified (in the recruitment process) and developed (via training and support). The challenge is to engender in advocates a sense of *intellectual independence*, that is, a sense in which loyalty to the client/partner, and a commitment to justice and empowerment, are paramount. Although ultimately rewarding, the process of advocacy is fraught with moral and ethical challenges which can overwhelm even the most enthusiastic social activist. How can advocacy schemes provide an environment in which this commitment is not only an aspiration, but realised and sustained?

Even within structurally independent schemes, the temptation for advocates to collude with service systems rather than remain loyal to their partners is all too real. Advocacy can sometimes be a lonely pastime, with few opportunities for positive feedback or information sharing. Against this backdrop, advocates may find themselves seduced by the camaraderie that often exists within large service provider organisations, or lured by the trappings of professionalisation. This is a failing of the advocacy movement as much as of the individual advocate. Speaking up for disempowered individuals, often within a hostile environment is a high–stress activity and advocates may seek support from wherever it is most readily available. If the advocacy schemes themselves have adequate support systems for their staff and volunteers then such problems would not arise. Support can be offered in the form of training, regular supervision and appraisal, team meetings and 'open door' access to senior project staff. It is also desirable that advocates have access to local support networks, which provide a useful forum for sharing experiences with other advocates and can help foster a sense of group identity unique to those involved with advocacy.

Equity

Throughout its history the provision and availability of advocacy for a wide range of potential beneficiaries has been sporadic, often based more on the individual interests of those developing services than on real local need. Up until very recently advocacy has too often been seen as a fringe activity or an expensive luxury as opposed to a key piece in the community care jigsaw. As a result, it has developed in a piecemeal manner, dependent on local and national trends in funding, opportunistic bidding or occasionally in response to crises and scandals in local service provision. It is surprisingly rare that advocacy services are developed as a result of strategic planning at a local (still less a national) level. The result is an inconsistent pattern of advocacy delivery that must be bewildering for potential users. Not only are different client groups served differently, but users also have the different advocacy forms to contend with. This situation is exacerbated by the fact that there exists no logical or systematic method of deciding which advocacy model is most appropriate in which situations. Consider the following example:

Area 1 (urban)

Citizen advocacy for over-65s living in residential care

Paid advocacy for people with mental health problems

Volunteer crisis advocacy for homeless Afro-Caribbeans

Area 2 (urban)

Paid advocacy for over-65s, carers and disabled people

Citizen advocacy for people with learning disabilities

Peer advocacy for young people looked after

Area 3 (rural)

No advocacy provision

Although it could be argued that inconsistencies such as those illustrated above could be resolved with effective strategic planning, this begs the question, whose responsibility is this? Most people within the advocacy movement would resist any moves seen to be imposing a uniform structure and code of practice on their activities. This is a key dichotomy – on the one hand needing to be independent, free from conflict of interest, grassroots, radical and locally accountable, and on the other wanting official recognition and status, long-term security and national influence. Much of the current debate within the national advocacy movement centres on this fundamental dilemma. There are those within the movement who claim that some advocacy (however patchy) is better than no advocacy; it is the responsibility of local communities to represent the needs of local devalued people. On this view, the impetus for advocacy should emerge not from the strategic plan of some bureaucratic agency but from social clubs, churches and workplaces. In other words, local people should promote the interests of local people – care *in* the community, *by* the community. If advocacy should grow from the grassroots, then equity cannot mean universal access imposed via 'top down' advocacy strategies – rather, it would mean fostering provision that meets the disadvantages of a particular area. In reality, however, it is often advocacy schemes themselves that bang the drum for more comprehensive advocacy provision in local areas. This dilemma is vividly illustrated below.

Planning advocacy provision

The local health authority wishes to commission advocacy for people living with HIV and AIDS. They contact all the existing advocacy schemes in their area and invite them to a meeting to discuss how the advocacy scheme might be run, and who would be best placed to run it.

"We believe that a Citizen Advocacy model would be most appropriate," says the coordinator of the local citizen advocacy scheme, "given that HIV is a long-term condition and hence people would be best served by a long-term, one-to-one relationship."

"And where do you expect to find volunteers who are willing to identify in a very personal way with a condition as stigmatising as HIV?," says the manager of a professional casework advocacy project. "It would be more efficient to recruit a team of advocacy workers who could work with larger numbers of people, dealing with crises as they arise."

"You are all missing the point," replies the peer advocacy project worker. "People with HIV need to be supported by people who themselves have been through the system. The most effective approach would be peer advocacy."

"My view is that whatever model we choose, the best provider would be an agency already well-established in the field, who has a proven track record in running a wide range of support services for this client group," says the director of a large service provider organisation. "That way, we can integrate advocacy with other local service provision."

Another feature of this dilemma is the extent to which existing advocacy provision is able to engage with all sections of the local community, and in particular with people from black and minority ethnic backgrounds. Much of the available research suggests that people from minority ethnic communities have an especially difficult time trying to obtain relevant services, either because such culturally appropriate services do not exist, or because mainstream services are insensitive to their needs. In a mental health context, there appears to be an even more serious problem. Not only are people from minority ethnic communities less likely to be offered beneficial treatments such as counselling and psychotherapy, they are more likely to be on the receiving end of coercive treatments like electroconvulsive therapy (ECT), high levels of psychiatric medication, seclusion and restraint (Fernando, 1991). Black people, especially young black men, are much more likely to be sectioned under the Mental Health Act than others (Francis et al, 1989; Bebbington et al, 1994). This represents a serious civil and human rights issue and is something that many mental health advocacy schemes are committed to challenging either on a one-to-one or group basis.

As advocacy is generally considered to be most appropriate when the needs and wishes of an individual or group are likely to be dismissed (Robson, 1987), it could be argued that people from ethnic minorities are in even greater need of advocacy, and one could expect that an even greater proportion of advocacy scheme clients will be from minority ethnic communities. Rogers and Pilgrim (1996, ch 7) endorse the Mental Health Task Force's conclusion that the provision of independent advocacy may be one way to improve mental health services for the black community. Francis et al (1989) also call for both legal and 'clinical' advocacy to be made available to people from ethnic minorities. However, in order for this to happen advocacy agencies need to be both *accessible and credible* to all sections of the local population. Equal opportunity is not only a goal for advocates to pursue, it is a principle which all schemes must embody. Although accessibility should be achievable, for example by ensuring publicity materials are available in different languages and formats and by organising open days targeted at particular minority communities, the issue of credibility is more complex. In order to appear credible to minority ethnic communities, to a degree that would encourage people to make use of advocacy, a number of criteria would need to be satisfied.

Availability. The extent to which the service is accessible and available to minority communities. Is the office base in an accessible building used by multiple communities? Does the scheme provide outreach to local groups and community buildings? Do local minority groups know about the scheme, via publicity, word of mouth, local networks?

Sensitivity. How does the service respond to enquiries from minority communities? Are there black and minority ethnic advocates available? Have all advocates had training on issues of race and culture? Is the scheme flexible and person-centred?

Language and cultural awareness. Do advocates and advocacy staff speak community languages? Does the scheme have a procedure for using interpreters? Are publicity materials available in different languages? Does the scheme work collaboratively with local minority community groups?

Anti-racist values and practices. Does the scheme have a workable equal opportunities policy? Where are job vacancies advertised? Does the scheme regularly review its core principles and practices? Are advocates given proper support and access to training?

Structural and intellectual independence. Is the scheme autonomous and free from conflicts of interest? Does the scheme have a local presence, and is it locally controlled? Are people from minority communities actively involved in the management and development of the scheme? Do advocates act in an independent and client-instructed way?

Loyalty

As previously stated, advocacy is often most effective when targeted at the least visible, least vocal, most vulnerable people in our communities. The UK advocacy movement has developed largely in response to the needs of users of community care services (older people, people with physical and sensory disabilities or mental health problems, people with learning disabilities, carers) and children and young people in care. The shared experience of many such people, especially those who have experienced periods of institutionalisation, is frequently one of disempowerment and discrimination. A central tenet of citizen advocacy philosophy is that devalued people (such as those described above) can derive some benefit from an organised 'matching' with ordinary citizens who are prepared to engage in a long-term, mutually beneficial relationship with them. The powerful testimony contained in *Standing by me* (Williams, 1998) proves that such partnerships can have a profound effect on the lives of both advocate and partner. Here is an example:

> My partner had quite a large sum of money at his nephew's and money in his flat, which concerned me as he was so vulnerable. I arranged an appointment with a local bank, and went with my partner to open a savings account where he could pay in his money.

All this was done under the wishes of my partner, who agreed it was a good idea. As my partner became anxious when attending appointments, I attended two doctor's appointments with him at his local GP surgery. There was a Care Plan meeting at a local hospital along with a review for my partner, and the social worker invited us both along, which I thought was very good of them. I really enjoy being a citizen advocate and find it very stimulating and rewarding. (Williams, 1998, p 30)

Clearly, both the advocate and partner in this vignette benefit from this relationship. On the one hand, the partner gains a confidante and representative who is prepared to take positive action to further his wishes and concerns, and on the other the advocate feels able to make a difference in the life of another citizen. While it is unhelpful to generalise on the possible motivation of people who act as advocates voluntarily, the desire to give back to the community is clearly an important driving force. By allying themselves in such a proactive way with devalued people, advocates challenge deeply held beliefs within society that reinforce the gulf between mad and sane, disabled and non-disabled, rich and poor. In so doing, they are contributing towards the development of a more tolerant society and a more caring community.

The loyalty that an advocate owes to their partner can be effective in a number of ways, then. At its root, however, it means 'being on the side' of the partner in an unambiguous way. The rationale for such a partial approach to supporting individuals is that the advocate remains untainted by external concerns and pressures. For example, an advocate can represent their partner's wish for additional hours of home support without concession to the resource problems of the local authority. This is not the same as being ignorant of such constraints, nor is it (as has sometimes been suggested) arrogance or belligerence. It is simply that the advocate's primary role is that of the 'voice' of the person in need. There are any number of other professionals, and sometimes family members, who are quick to assume the mantle of advisor, mediator or gatekeeper. The decision about whether to award the extra care hours is not the advocate's – but an effective advocate will ensure that their partner's views have been clearly represented and positively received.

Thus, a commitment to the individual and to the advocate and partner relationship remains a fundamental principle of contemporary advocacy. Without such a commitment, there would be a very real danger that advocacy becomes just another service, providing advice or a version of social work. Some commentators have openly suggested that the future of advocacy lies in pursuing just such objectives. Atkinson (1999) clearly identifies informal social work as a possible way forward for advocacy, in addition to helping to safeguard people from abuse and neglect (see Chapter Three for a more detailed analysis of this work). How far can the intangible but powerful quality of loyalty be codified in a series of 'interventions'? The answer given to this question will indeed shape the future of advocacy provision; it will be a key aim of this book to provide some sort of answer to this question.

However, it is sometimes argued that by focusing exclusively on loyalty to the individual, advocacy denies the collective experience of disempowerment and more importantly, the collective experience of empowerment that is such a key feature of the service user movement. For example, Bateman (2000) argues that:

> Advocacy can also be limited in its effects by being too closely linked with individualism. Most of the problems which advocates resolve will be faced by hundreds of thousands of other people. Not only can advocacy take on a collective form, but it is more effective if used as part of a wider strategy for helping others. (Bateman, 2000, p 181)

Organisations such as People First, Survivors Speak Out and the Direct Action Network have enabled users to join together to challenge inequalities and campaign for improved service provision and greater recognition of peoples' civil and human rights. Although the methodology may differ, most user groups share the common aims of encouraging people to take pride in their identity and campaigning for a change in attitude towards disabled people. This collective approach is in contrast to the individualistic model adopted within advocacy. The advocacy and user movements can be seen as allied and complementary rather than unified, although there are strong links between user groups and the concept of self-advocacy. Whether advocacy schemes could and should do more to align themselves with the user movement will be considered in Chapters Five and Six.

Risk

Whenever the term 'community care' is used these days, it seems that 'risk management' will follow with the next breath. Whereas, 20 years ago, scandals concerning the abuse of patients helped to seal the fate of the long-stay hospitals, now media attention seems to play a much more ambivalent role. Tragic instances of killings by individuals with mental health problems have created a perception of this group as presenting an undue risk to the public, and therefore needing closer 'supervision'. Even where service users themselves are the victims of crime, this tends to be blamed on a lack of 'support' from service providers, rather than on the criminality of the perpetrator.

It is small wonder, then, that services have felt the need to adopt strategies which aim to protect both users and the public, and to defend themselves against litigation or public criticism. It is equally unsurprising that service users and their advocates have viewed this double agenda as potentially undermining of individual freedom and development. Risk management appears to restore to the 'medical model' of care much of the power and prestige it lost when care in the community was first implemented.

Yet if the advocacy movement is rightly wary of risk management, it cannot afford to ignore the question of individual vulnerability either. How does an advocate or scheme respond if a partner discloses abuse? What steps do schemes take to ensure that abusers do not become advocates? How can an advocate help someone who has severe learning difficulties and mental health problems to discover positive opportunities if they do not know what circumstances are likely to make that person anxious or unwell? How do schemes deal with the possibility that they may be the objects of litigation by dissatisfied partners or advocates? If any of these questions require credible, sustainable answers – and we believe they all do – then advocacy schemes need at least some systems by which they can assess and respond to risk. There are three main areas where a form of risk assessment may be appropriate:

- risk to the advocate
- risk to the partner
- risk to the advocacy relationship.

Risk to the advocate. To the extent that advocates like many others are operating at the 'front line' then they are at risk of violence and aggression from people who may be unhappy with the way they have been treated within service systems. Although advocates identify clearly with the views and concerns of their partners, there will be times when the advocacy role is not well understood and the advocate is perceived to be part of 'the system'. In addition, there are inherent risks associated with any form of outreach work which involves visiting people in their own homes, especially in the early stages of an advocacy relationship when boundaries are not yet negotiated or agreed. Another potential risk is that partners may develop unrealistic expectations of what their advocate will be able to achieve, and become disappointed if progress is not as quick or comprehensive as they would like. It is therefore incumbent on schemes to ensure that advocates are briefed and supported in the process of risk assessment without raising undue concern or fear.

Risk to the partner. By this we mean risk from the advocates themselves, whether in the form of physical, financial or emotional abuse. Although most advocacy schemes adopt stringent recruitment and selection processes (and many require police checks on their advocates), there will still be occasions where an unscrupulous individual 'slips through the net' and goes on to abuse their position of trust for their own ends. In such a situation, the advocacy scheme needs to be able to demonstrate it has the capacity and will to learn from its mistakes and take swift action to avoid any repetition of events. Advocacy partners should also be given easy access to complaints procedures and to scheme managers or coordinators in order to minimise the risk of a 'culture of secrecy' emerging within both advocacy partnerships and the wider scheme.

Risk to the advocacy relationship. By its very nature, advocacy exists to challenge inequalities and highlight areas of bad practice or neglect. In so doing, advocates and their partners run the risk of being targeted or threatened by the perpetrators of such acts. This is particularly true in institutionalised or segregated settings where there is a large social control element to the environment or culture. Advocates, like 'whistleblowers', have been victim to threats and assaults as a result of their role in exposing malpractice on behalf of their partners. There may be a potential role for codes of practice for advocacy which place value on the advocacy role and outline measures to safeguard advocates and partners from such intimidation.

How to evaluate advocacy?

There is currently no widely accepted standard framework for monitoring and regulating advocacy in the UK. Although the United Kingdom Advocacy Network's (UKAN) *Advocacy: A Code of Practice* (UKAN, 1997) and the type of code suggested by Citizen Advocacy Information and Training (Wertheimer, 1998) are influential in their respective fields, neither has been adopted as comprehensively as some may have wanted. Local advocacy initiatives have developed largely autonomously with their own identities, procedures and monitoring arrangements. While this has undoubtedly led to more localised and informal arrangements for users, the problem of how best to promote and monitor effectiveness remains. In the absence of agreed standards the monitoring agenda has increasingly been set by funding agencies, who often have little knowledge or regard for the particular aims and methods of advocacy schemes. The tendency to fall back on tried and tested quantitative measures means that the intrinsic value of advocacy – the stories of advocates and partners, the quest for social change and justice – often goes unmeasured and hence unrecognised. This is not to say that advocacy schemes should be exempted from any monitoring or regulatory requirements: if schemes are accepting public money, they should be prepared to be held to account for how that money is spent. The issue is about *how* advocacy programmes are most appropriately measured rather than *if* they should be. In subsequent chapters it will be argued that traditional 'service' measures do not provide sufficient depth or sensitivity truly to demonstrate the worth of advocacy in the lives of disempowered people.

Although schemes will certainly aspire to having basic service standards and measures in place (waiting times, ethnic monitoring, complaints procedures and so on), they also need to develop the means to provide some evidence of the more cerebral and empowering aspects of advocacy. At the very least these should include some evidence of effective advocate/partner matching processes (based, for example, on factors such as common interests, skills match, cultural and language needs); the minimisation of dependency and maximisation of empowerment; a focus on outcomes as well as processes; and a commitment to equality of opportunity.

It is clear that a qualitative approach to data collection will be required in order to obtain the appropriate information as outlined above. There are a number of factors which conspire to make such data collection problematic in an advocacy context. For example, there is a lack of agreement as to what constitutes effective advocacy. The concept of advocacy is still a relatively new one, and levels of knowledge about advocacy among the general public are poor. There is no clearly defined frame of reference by which people can judge whether the advocacy support they receive is 'good' or 'bad'. When a customer goes into a high street burger bar they have a very good idea of what to expect – what the burger will look and taste like, how it will be packaged, how much it will cost. There are no such easily quantifiable standards for advocacy and hence, no simple way of comparing peoples experiences of advocacy to a set of pre-determined and consistent standards.

Is there then a place for national standards in regulating advocacy provision? On the one hand, the vulnerability of some of those supported by advocates (people with dementia, those who have experienced abuse) suggests that some common safeguards are required. On the other hand, the diversity of advocacy forms, and their jealous guarding of advocacy practice, suggests that such standards may be impossible to develop. Chapter Six will pursue this question further.

Similar questions arise in relation to the training of advocates. If advocacy is a skill, it should be possible to develop and refine it through training. On this view, the accreditation of advocates through, say, National Vocational Qualifications (NVQs) seems a possible, even a desirable course. If, however, advocacy is primarily about one person's commitment to another's cause, training will be at best a secondary issue. The subject of training is explored in more detail in Chapter Seven.

A key question in both the opening chapter and this has been 'What constitutes good advocacy?' If the advocacy movement is serious in its pursuit of secure funding, if it is concerned to maintain a coherent values-base for advocacy practice, it must be able to answer this question. Mechanisms for evaluating advocacy will have a central place in any such answer; and it is with the question of evaluation that the next chapter is concerned.

THREE

Problems in measuring advocacy outcomes

In Chapter One, a lack of identity, coherence and consistency were identified as obstacles to the continued development of the advocacy movement in the UK. Chapter Two looked at the ways in which this overall lack of stability placed question marks over key advocacy principles such as independence and loyalty. Yet these problems exist against a backdrop of dynamism, growth and well-attested success within the advocacy movement. How – in the jargon of the business world – can the advocacy movement marshal its strengths to counter its weaknesses?

Dorothy Atkinson's *Advocacy: A review* (1999) seeks to undertake the first part of this task: to establish a baseline for existing advocacy provisions, and to suggest ways of developing them. This work gives a good outline of the different types of advocacy schemes that operate in the UK. Atkinson's fieldwork provides ample evidence that:

> Advocacy is an empowering process ... this applies across its many manifestations, from supportive self advocacy groups, through peer advocacy schemes, to citizen advocacy, and advocacy provided by paid sessional and full-time workers. (Atkinson, 1999, p 22)

This finding could be a springboard for the development of an advocacy movement diverse in its practices yet unified around the central concept of empowerment. But this is unlikely to happen.

> One of the things that stops advocacy from working effectively is the internal division about what it is, who does it and who it is for.... Some disabled people see citizen advocacy in its pure form as potentially a devaluing process in itself. (Atkinson, 1999, p 25)

To cite one example of these divisions: the citizen advocacy model is seen to hinge on the provision of 'valued citizens' to advocate for apparently 'devalued' partners. Some disabled people see this as simply reinforcing perceptions that they are invariably 'needy' or 'dependent', never able or empowered. Needless to say, the citizen advocacy movement emphatically rejects this criticism; it sees advocacy partnerships as the best way to *challenge* these false perceptions. Yet the disagreement could hardly be more profound: what one side sees as the *answer* is seen by the other as a further *problem*.

Whether or not there is a right answer here, the argument shows that the advocacy movement clearly has problems in establishing a purely descriptive baseline for advocacy practice. Advocacy processes appear to be inseparable from the value-claims made for them. Thus, John O'Brien's definition of citizen advocacy is also a claim for its results, describing:

> A valued citizen ... bringing their partner's gifts and concerns into the circles of ordinary community life. (O'Brien, quoted in Atkinson, 1999, p 7)

Similarly, Atkinson's own definition of peer advocacy describes both the process and the anticipated result, as though they were almost the same thing:

> The advocate in this instance is an insider, someone who is in the know through personal experience of disability or mental health problems, and so can draw on that experience to show empathy and understanding. (Atkinson, 1999, p 7)

Time and again in advocacy one comes across this blurring of aims (*what* an advocacy scheme is trying to achieve) and principles (the rules describing *how* a scheme will go about achieving its aims). When Atkinson writes that advocacy is about empowerment, autonomy, citizenship and inclusion (1999, p 16), it is clear that these are not only the *benefits* it aims to bring, but also the *kinds of practice* which any credible scheme should follow. It is as though there is something exemplary about the advocate's role; they are not just deploying various tactics in order to get a result for their partner, they are developing a particular kind of *relationship* with that person, one which is meant to change and inspire the way that others relate to them. The blurring of aims and principles marks advocacy out as an arena which aspires to commitment, conviction, and direct social change.

Yet if this blurring shows the strong ideals (and high expectations) which lie behind advocacy, it is also a breeding ground for confusion within the advocacy movement. It is all too easy for advocacy schemes to assume that because their aims are worthy, and their practice principled, valid outcomes must inevitably be achieved. To return to the argument between citizen and peer advocacy cited above, there is an assumption in each case that because the advocate has something plausible to offer ('valued' status in the case of the citizen advocate, solidarity in the case of the peer), this will *necessarily* be transmitted as a benefit to the advocacy partner. But this is not so; in either case, any one of a dozen factors could neutralise this potential benefit. The advocate, for all their apparent suitability as a citizen or peer, may lack sufficient commitment to their role – or the partner may simply not like them. The advocate may not have the skills required for a particular situation, or may be inadequately supported. To put it another way, an advocacy scheme may be principled without necessarily being effective. While a certain blurring of aims and principles may be a hallmark of true advocacy, the confusion of aims with results should be challenged.

If principles alone cannot measure the impact of individual advocacy schemes, this task must be completed by evaluation. Interestingly, although it contains much feedback from users of advocacy, *Advocacy: A review* (Atkinson, 1999) is virtually silent on the subject of formal evaluation. This silence detracts from the author's otherwise valid call for the development of an 'advocacy culture' – a key concept which will be more fully explored in Chapter Five. Evaluation which links principles, practice and outcomes and generates evidence which can inform practitioners, users, funders and others, should be the bedrock of this culture. Without it, attempts to promote advocacy as a whole will founder amid the competing and unverified claims made for the principles and relative merits of different types of schemes.

Atkinson's own conclusions and recommendations are in fact somewhat disappointing in their lack of confidence in the distinctive nature of advocacy. She rightly observes that,

> ... advocacy often means more than supporting people to have a say in their lives, it means supporting them in managing their lives. (Atkinson, 1999, p 34)

But this does not entirely warrant her description of advocacy as 'the reinvention of social work'. Social work is society's intervention, however benign, in the life of the individual; advocacy gives the individual the right to intervene in and to change social and service processes. Again, Atkinson correctly asserts that: "advocacy has the potential to protect people from abuse" (p 35), but her statement that children's advocacy (seemingly because of its use of professionals as advocates and more rigorous procedures) has most to offer in this respect seems arbitrary. Are not other kinds of advocacy also effective in preventing abuse? In fact, it might be argued that the best 'watchdogs' of services prone to commit abusive or unethical practices are those *without* a professional background and hence free from the preconceptions which come from years of working in human service settings.

The lack of a clear evaluative framework undermines the attempt to develop the concept of an advocacy culture and, arguably, leaves Atkinson's recommendations for the future of advocacy too close to social work models. But her lack of reference to evaluation is understandable if one recognises that there are currently very few designated models of advocacy evaluation. The main ones are considered below.

Citizen Advocacy Program Evaluation

Citizen Advocacy Program Evaluation (CAPE) was developed by John O'Brien and Wolf Wolfensberger (1979) in the late 1970s. It was subsequently complemented by O'Brien's *Learning from citizen advocacy programs* (1987). CAPE comprehensively defines the principles of citizen advocacy, and requires the evaluator to rate a scheme's success in implementing each principle, usually on a scale of 1 to 4, with 1 pointing to "major deficiencies in complying with the principle of the rating" with 4 denoting "distinctly positive implementation" (O'Brien and Wolfensberger, 1979, p 3). The ratings are given their impetus above all by the authors' demand that citizen advocacy be as unlike 'human services' (care services) as possible. The independence of advocacy schemes is upheld, not only so that advocates can act freely, but also so that the scheme does not look or feel like a care service. Advocates must have a primary loyalty to their partner in order to speak with conviction on their behalf, and to avoid the advocacy office becoming the dominant player in the relationship; becoming, that is, a 'human service'. Twenty years on, it is easy to forget how radical this rejection of the service approach was and is. For O'Brien and Wolfensberger, the crucial first step in the defence and promotion of people's rights is the establishment of relationships based on conviction, not money. In place of paid care services which are seen as segregating, stigmatising and controlling, they propose an advocacy which is freely given, open-ended and inclusive. CAPE is therefore intended not only as a positive record of advocacy implementation; it is also seen as an enduring safeguard against the possibility of advocacy being taken over by a hostile service culture.

CAPE is still used by UK citizen advocacy schemes, although there are perhaps only one or two such evaluations each year. CAPE's strengths are several. First, it establishes the importance of the links between principles and practice in advocacy, and provides tools for assessing and developing these links. Second, it provides (if used by a qualified evaluator) an objective measure of a scheme's performance against a set of constant standards. Finally, it highlights the way in which evaluation can – and should – be an integral part of a developing advocacy culture which is entirely distinct from service models.

But there are a number of difficulties surrounding CAPE, too, which perhaps explain why it is relatively little used. First, there are cultural difficulties in CAPE for UK schemes. For instance, to score even a satisfactory level 3 rating, a scheme is required by CAPE to have 60-80% of its funding from non-service funders *and* its funding should come from three to five different funding sources. In a country where corporate and charitable trust giving lags far behind the US, and local government has traditionally been the only core funding agency for local voluntary groups (while providing many care services of its own), this seems a tall order. CAPE's ratings system can appear to 'punish' schemes for cultural and political conditions which lie far beyond their control.

Second, and crucially, CAPE does not offer any measure of or comment on a scheme's impact. Even *Learning from citizen advocacy programs*, while offering guidelines for interviewing advocacy partnerships, admits that it:

> ... says little about the wide variety of things people in citizen advocacy relationships actually do together. (O'Brien, 1987, p 1)

This reticence is understandable. The citizen advocacy partnership should be owned by advocate and partner, not by the scheme. A citizen advocate does not have to 'report back' to their scheme in order to have their activity validated or assessed. Nonetheless, silence on the subject of impact means that a CAPE evaluation is unlikely to promote the value of a scheme's endeavours to the sceptical. It will be of limited use in showing funders how their money is being spent. CAPE's audience may in the final analysis be a fairly narrow one, consisting primarily of advocacy movement 'insiders'.

At worst CAPE could (and perhaps has) contributed to the development of a climate in which a scheme's 'purity' (its adherence to principle) is taken as a guarantee of its effectiveness in helping its partners. Such assumptions are not justified: principles may be *essential*, they are not *sufficient*. There is a danger here of elitism, of placing theoretical proficiency ahead of the core citizen advocacy values of inclusiveness and relationship.

Finally, CAPE is, by definition, only an evaluation of citizen advocacy schemes. Other types of scheme may gain insights from it, but could not be evaluated by it. Indeed, CAPE seeks to distance citizen advocacy from other types of advocacy almost as much as it does from 'human services':

> Clear and effective staff functioning requires … non-competition with other advocacy roles. (O'Brien and Wolfsenberger, 1979, p 10)

Granted the need for clarity, one still wonders if there are not valid and informative questions to be asked about how a citizen advocacy scheme relates to other advocacy schemes in its locality. The citizen advocacy movement could offer counter-arguments to each of these points, and it is true that the criticisms may be a matter of perception as much as of substance. But perceptions matter; in order to fulfil its role, an evaluatory system must be credible to *all* interested parties.

None of this is to deny that CAPE has been, and continues to be, a source of inspiration for citizen advocacy in the UK. Its standards are a touchstone for schemes even if they cannot comply with all of them, and CAPE evaluations have been an effective developmental tool for the schemes they have covered. Our review has suggested that there may need to be evaluatory mechanisms for citizen advocacy in addition to CAPE. Such is the remit of the CAIT evaluation pack described below.

CAIT evaluation pack

Citizen Advocacy Information and Training (CAIT) produced its evaluation pack in 1998, after a considerable period of consultation with citizen advocacy schemes (Hanley and Davies, 1998). The pack addresses two of the difficulties in CAPE: the sometimes arbitrary system of ratings and the lack of information about advocacy partnership activity. The CAIT pack sets out the same citizen advocacy principles as CAPE, but allows for the fact that individual schemes may not aspire to meet all of these standards all of the time. Local conditions may make different aims necessary or desirable. Schemes are therefore measured against their own aims, as well as against citizen advocacy principles.

A CAIT evaluation team will seek to meet with eight citizen advocates and their partners within a given scheme as part of the evaluation process. The purpose of these meetings is not to evaluate the partnerships themselves, but to gain from them an understanding of how the scheme is working in practice. By interviewing partnerships, the evaluator can begin to identify, for example:

- the range of people the scheme is helping
- the types of role advocates are taking on (for example, friend, negotiator, information gatherer etc)
- how well the scheme has prepared advocates for their role
- how far advocates are loyal to their partners, rather than to the scheme.

Thus, when used by trained evaluators, the CAIT pack should convey not only technical information about the meeting of aims and standards, but something of the 'feel' of an advocacy scheme.

However, in interviewing advocacy partnerships, the CAIT pack still basically adheres to the idea that to act in a principled way is to be a successful advocate:

> We believe that the process of citizen advocacy is important and valuable in itself, over and above 'outcomes'. (Hanley and Davies, 1998, p 17)

Certainly, it would be entirely inappropriate to form judgements about individual citizen advocacy partnerships; as freely given relationships, these cannot be measured against a common standard any more than people can. Confidentiality, too, is a barrier to gaining a full picture of a scheme's activity from its partnerships: a partner who has been helped through a traumatic, personal crisis by their advocate is unlikely to expose themselves to interview, yet their partnership may be one of the scheme's most significant outcomes. Still, the CAIT pack does not really generate a sense of the scheme's overall impact. Partnerships do not have to be evaluated, but the evidence gained from them could perhaps be 'joined up' in some way. Does the evidence say something about the ways in which the scheme is influencing the local community, or local services, for instance?

Like CAPE, the CAIT evaluation system seems to be addressed primarily to advocacy 'insiders'. The introduction talks of its role in

> ... encouraging schemes to feel positive about what's going well, and learn more about how they can improve more difficult areas. (Hanley and Davies, 1998, p 3)

If advocacy was universally seen to be a worthwhile activity, and citizen advocacy was agreed to be the pre-eminent model, this approach might be sufficient. But neither is the case. All of the bodies who fund citizen advocacy (be it local government, the National Lottery [now called Community Fund] or charitable trusts) face large and competing demands on their resources; should not evaluation assure them that their money is being spent, not only on a principled and competent organisation, but also on a significant and effective activity?

Nor is it only funders who may need to be educated and persuaded by advocacy evaluation. User groups, carers, ratepayers and even the services with whom advocates come into contact may all have differing kinds of interest in what an advocacy scheme is doing, and how well it is doing it. Perhaps some of these groups should be represented within the evaluation process. Talking to a service manager *might* shed light on a scheme's activity. Of course, he or she may simply wish to denigrate a scheme that is asking awkward questions of their service, but a well-structured interview should expose such agendas.

The CAIT evaluation pack, then, has much to recommend it, but still poses three problems:

- it is heavily focused on principles, at the expense of outcomes
- it is addressed primarily to others within the advocacy movement
- it is only designed for citizen advocacy schemes.

ANNETTE

Three years before the publication of the CAIT evaluation pack, a very different evaluation appeared, which anticipated and sought to tackle head-on the three problems set out above. 'ANNETTE', the Advocacy Network Newcastle (ANN) evaluation tool (ANN, 1995), sought to make an advocacy scheme's principles subordinate to its *goal achievement*. It sets out tables for recording any issues which an advocate has helped their partner to identify, raise or resolve during the period under review. The issues are counted up and, though there is a place for commentary on some of these, it is the numerical tally that is the primary measure of the scheme's impact. As the authors write:

> We wanted to develop quantitative measures for the qualitative change brought about through advocacy. (ANN, 1995, p 7)

The impetus for this radical approach comes from ANNETTE's intended audience. Whereas CAPE and the CAIT pack are addressed primarily to those within the advocacy movement,

> ANNETTE was developed in response to the needs of purchasers who wanted to be sure that the *effectiveness* of advocacy could be measured to ensure that they were getting value for money". (ANN, 1995, p 7)

And although ANNETTE is designed to be compatible with citizen advocacy principles, it could just as easily be used by schemes offering short-term or professional advocacy. For advocacy processes too are measured, not in terms of principles, but in terms of numbers. Types of advocacy role are grouped under six headings ('mediator', 'trouble shooter', 'special friend', 'confidant', 'guide', and 'lifeguard') and the number of advocates taking on each type of role are added up. ANNETTE also records the number of hours given by advocates during the review period as a further indicator of process.

ANNETTE envisages an advocacy culture that is driven by outputs and outcomes. It holds out to advocacy schemes of all kinds the prospect of straightforwardly measuring, and demonstrating, their impact. A corollary of this, of course, is that schemes could also be compared with each other using standards derived from ANNETTE, with some being judged better than others. The world of outputs and outcomes is also the world of competition.

The service culture and Best Value

There are significant problems with the ANNETTE approach, which will shortly be discussed. But whatever its shortcomings as an evaluation tool (and it does not seem to have been widely used by advocacy schemes) ANNETTE's authors clearly understood the funding and monitoring environment in which the advocacy movement found itself at the end of the 20th century. The key fact here is that the majority of UK advocacy schemes are, as Chapter Two showed, core funded by local authorities (and to a lesser extent, the NHS). The most obvious problem this creates is potential conflict of interest; an advocacy scheme that is funded by a social services department may find it difficult to challenge the actions of that department. Or, if they do challenge, they may face the withdrawal of their funding.

Conflict of interest poses a real threat to the independence and effectiveness of advocacy schemes. But it is arguably not the greatest threat associated with current advocacy funding arrangements. This comes from the whole service culture in which local authorities and the NHS now operate. The roots of this culture lie in the revolution which swept through industry in the 1980s. Where previously the commercial and political worlds had been preoccupied with concerns about the *production* of goods, with questions about industrial strategy and workers' rights to the fore, the Thatcher era saw these concerns replaced by a single-minded focus on meeting the needs of the *consumer*. The same shift saw the competing ideologies of the industrial era displaced by the 'post-ideological' concept of the 'service'.

This revolution in outlook was introduced to the public sector in the 1990s. Its guiding principle was quality, and its effects were felt in a much more directive managerial culture, and in the introduction of compulsory competitive tendering. Providers of services no longer held that status as of right; the fact that they were doing something 'worthwhile in itself' (as the CAIT evaluation pack describes citizen advocacy) counted for nothing, unless they could show that they were doing it more efficiently and more effectively than other providers. Not only local authorities themselves, but also the voluntary organisations that they funded, were caught up in the demands of the

Figure 1: The service model

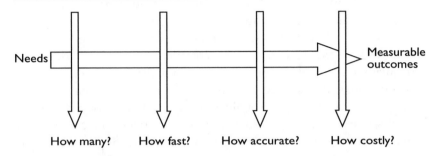

'contract culture'. If we were to try to model this culture as it affects the provision of community and welfare activities, it might look something like the above (see Figure 1).

There are two key concerns for an organisation following this model. The first is that it should be achieving demonstrable results or outcomes, and the second is that it should be achieving these with maximum efficiency: as many as possible, as quickly as possible, as accurately as possible, for the least cost possible. In its current political form, this is the culture of 'Best Value'.

Best Value is defined by the 1999 Local Government Act which requires local authorities to,

> Secure continuous improvement in the way in which they exercise their functions, having regard to a combination of economy, efficiency and effectiveness. (DETR, 1999, p 3)

In order to meet this requirement, local authorities must undertake Best Value reviews of all their services, whether they provide these directly or purchase them from independent provider agencies. Underpinning all such reviews are four key principles:

- *challenging* why and how a service is being provided
- *comparing* performance with that of other similar services
- *consulting* service users and taxpayers to set new targets
- using the principles of 'fair *competition*' in deciding who should provide the service.

It is not the purpose of this book to attempt to evaluate Best Value culture as a whole; doubtless it has brought both gains and losses. What is important here is the impact it is having on advocacy provision.

As we noted above, ANNETTE is an evaluation tool which anticipates and is at home in a Best Value environment. It is pragmatic (it can accommodate a range of advocacy styles), it measures both process and benefit, and it allows comparison between schemes. Indeed, while ANNETTE was designed to be compliant with citizen advocacy principles, its emphasis on statistics means that in any comparative evaluation, a professional casework advocacy scheme which simply helped people through particular problems and then stopped working with them would be judged 'better' than a citizen advocacy scheme based on long-term partnerships that may go through spells where there are no obvious issues to address.

This does indeed appear to be the conclusion reached by many Best Value funders. While the recent growth of casework advocacy schemes and relative decline in the number of citizen advocacy schemes doubtless reflects a range of factors (for example user groups wishing to develop their own models), there can be little doubt that funders' perceptions have played a major role here. An extreme confirmation of this trend is given by the appearance in one or two parts of the UK of 'spot purchased' advocacy. Under this arrangement, there is no core funding provided for advocacy. Instead, social services managers make one-off payments to an advocacy provider whenever they determine that one of their clients needs an advocate. This approach has two significant implications; first, that local authorities become the gatekeepers for advocacy, removing much of its independence in the process, and second, that in the absence of core funding for agencies which concentrate their energies entirely on advocacy, advocacy could only be provided by organisations which gain their regular income from one or another form of service provision. It will be argued in Chapter Five that this trend undermines the provision of good advocacy. For now, it is sufficient to note that Best Value may not simply regulate advocacy; it may also alter its principles and practice.

Is this not a good thing? If one type of scheme achieves more results than another, and does so more efficiently, should not that type of scheme come to predominate? Put like this, the case seems unarguable. If, on the other hand, the Best Value approach is based on a mistaken assumption about what good advocacy is, and if in the making of that assumption, fundamental advocacy needs have been distorted or ignored, one would have to question the validity of this approach in evaluating advocacy.

There are, in fact, four grounds for challenging the Best Value approach adopted by ANNETTE and many scheme funders. These may be characterised as follows:

- the ambiguity of 'measurable outcomes'
- the preventive effects of advocacy
- difficulties in gaining user feedback
- the rationing agenda.

The ambiguity of 'measurable outcomes'

A key premise of ANNETTE is that an advocacy scheme's effectiveness can be measured by the extent to which it helps partners to achieve 'goals'; these equate to 'measurable outcomes' in the model in Figure 1. In the market system from which the Best Value approach draws much of its inspiration, outcomes are often easily monitored. If, for example, someone buys an insurance policy, they will judge it successful if they receive the correct amount of money when the insured event occurs, and if the company handling the claim is courteous and efficient.

It is tempting to think that advocacy outcomes would be similarly easy to pin down. Certainly, the language used by health and social services during the past 10 years and the proliferation of charters defining levels of service, suggest a provider–customer contract similar to the insurance purchase just described. Yet the outcomes these organisations aim at, and the processes through which they are to be achieved, are much more complex than commercial transactions. Health cannot be bought over the counter in a box, and exactly what constitutes 'helping disabled people to live independently in the community', for example, may be defined in a dozen different ways by 'consumers' and 'providers'. In these instances, it is much harder to provide unambiguous indicators of success.

The danger here is that *arbitrary* or *incomplete* criteria are used for judging the success of health or social care activities. A notorious illustration of this can be found in the NHS waiting lists initiatives launched by the government in the early 1990s. Here was a worthy objective, if ever there was one: that fewer people should wait less time for surgery. The means for reducing the waiting lists was the introduction of targets: no patient should wait longer than a certain period of time for surgery. Here, too, was apparent success: within months, waiting times had come down – the goals were being met.

Only slowly did it emerge that at least part of the reduction in waiting times was an illusion; many patients were now having to join 'unofficial' waiting lists before being put onto the official one. Similarly, an apparently impressive growth in the numbers of patients treated was at least partly accounted for by the fact that patients who had been discharged too soon from hospital (so that new patients could be admitted in order to meet waiting list targets) and then had to be re-admitted, were counted as 'new' patients. An apparent success masked a real and serious failure.

Doubtless, performance indicators within the NHS have undergone considerable refinement in the intervening years, but similar arguments persist. At the time of writing, the government is proclaiming its success in reducing *waiting lists*, while the opposition seeks to highlight an increase in *waiting times*. Our story highlights three potential problems for the use of 'measurable outcomes' in the social care sector:

- apparent success may not equal real success
- the use of targets may distort the very activity they are supposed to measure
- the goals or targets selected may reflect the needs of the funder (a government in need of 'good news' for example) rather than the needs of users.

Each of these points highlights difficulties for a model of advocacy that places too much emphasis on 'goal-achievement' as the measure of its success. It could be genuinely informative for an advocacy scheme to collate figures showing the number of partners it has helped with housing problems or benefits tribunals. But it would be misleading to try to set strict standards for success in terms of how many tenancies advocates have brokered, or how much additional benefit has been 'won'. An advocate might succeed in getting their partner discharged from a Mental Health Act section, but if that person is re-sectioned a few weeks later because too little thought was given to their after-care, what sort of success is this?

Second, there is a real danger that a scheme that focuses primarily on 'goal achievement' will tend to work primarily with those who are able to make their wishes known fairly readily. How, for example, would a goal-based scheme work with those who have severe learning disabilities or dementia? Would it create long-term partnerships with them, recognising that these may not produce 'results' for a long time? Or would it, under pressure to achieve outcomes, allow its advocates to act as arbitrators, substituting their views for those of the partner? Or indeed, would it simply not work with these groups at all? If it follows the latter options, are we not entitled to say that the scheme's work has been distorted by its pursuit of 'measurable outcomes', and that it is no longer working in an ethical way with those very disempowered groups who arguably have most need of advocacy? Comparing the effectiveness of different advocacy schemes, as the BestValue process envisages, seems sound in principle, but if the data on which the comparison is to be based are contrived or misleading, the process is worthless.

The preventive effects of advocacy

Roger

Roger had lived for many years in a long-stay institution. He moved to a group home eight years ago, where he used to respond to stress by banging his head or biting his wrist. He was introduced to a citizen advocate, Mark, and soon began to go out with him regularly. Mark encouraged Roger's interest in photography, and they built up a large scrapbook. Mark was careful to give Roger the final say on what went in the scrapbook. After about 18 months, Mark attended Roger's review meeting, where staff commented on the reduction in Roger's 'distress' behaviours. His medication was reduced as a result. Although Mark rarely spoke on Roger's behalf, he had helped him to feel much more certain of himself.

Protection

A professional advocate with a mental health scheme found she was getting many enquiries from residents in a group of private hostels who felt they had no control over their personal finances. Finally, she asked social services to investigate. No wrongdoing was proven, but within six months social services had issued a new code of conduct for service providers, and many more service users were able to set up their own bank accounts.

US citizen advocacy schemes have always referred to the people they support as 'protégés'. The term is not used in this country, perhaps because it is perceived as paternalistic or patronising. Yet the term contains one important truth that is anecdotally confirmed by many advocacy schemes: that the mere presence of an advocate within a given situation tips the balance of power at least some way back towards the person they represent. The two brief anecdotes cited above seem to highlight this sort of effect. In neither case is there a clear 'goal', but in each instance something important has undoubtedly happened. In Roger's case, he has probably been spared further physical pain and risk, and perhaps the need for psychological or medical treatment, but it cannot be proved that this was the result of advocacy. In the second story, entire service processes have changed, with benefits to many users, but there is no 'proven' link with the actions of the advocate.

The preventive effects of advocacy can perhaps only fully be articulated through stories like those given above; they cannot be reduced to a series of comparative indices.

Difficulties in gaining user feedback

Perhaps the most simple and direct way to evaluate a service – used by shops and public authorities alike – is to ask for the views of its customers. Consumer satisfaction is generally seen as one of an organisation's greatest assets, and the key indicator of its success. This is reflected in the BestValue guidance already quoted, which highlights the importance of consulting with service users. In some ways, it is surprising that the advocacy movement has not generated more in the way of systematic procedures for gaining comments and complaints from its users or partners. The tradition of telling partnership stories in citizen advocacy goes some way towards meeting this need, and *Standing by me* (Williams, 1998) gives many good examples of this, but still one wonders exactly how schemes are finding out, for example, whether partners are happy with their advocates and how they respond if the partners are not happy.

It seems likely that much more could be done to collect user feedback in a systematic way, and to use the evidence gained to improve advocacy practice. But here, too, a note of caution must be sounded. A complicating factor in attempting to collect accurate data about advocacy is what has become known as the 'halo' or 'hero' effect. People often approach advocacy schemes at the point at which their own efforts to resolve problems have failed. Approaching an advocacy scheme for help requires a great deal of courage, and a significant emotional and psychological investment on the part of the client/ partner. In order to justify this investment, clients/partners will sometimes go to great lengths to ascribe high status to their advocates, believing them to have special skills or 'inside information' which can be utilised on their behalf. Of course, there may be some truth in this (advocates often do have a great deal of experience in tackling issues) but, coupled with the fact that advocates are often described by clients/ partners as "the only person who listens to me", it is clear why some caution should be exercised in relation to analysing people's rating of their advocate's performance.

Of course, some advocacy partners can give very clear feedback. At the National Mind conference held in London in 1999, Dr Rachel Perkins, a mental health service user and psychologist, told the audience how she has drawn up a list of her needs, wishes and expectations for treatment when ill. When she becomes ill, her advocate's sole task is to ensure that this plan is implemented by the services responsible. Here the advocate's own views are very deliberately kept out of the picture. The advocate is, as it were, merely an instrument for ensuring that the partner's views are respected at a time when they otherwise might not be. Although the advocate's skills will be important in negotiating the plan with services, their *relationship* to the partner is immaterial. They are speaking up, not necessarily because they know her well (as a carer or relative might), but because the partner's wishes must be paramount. This is a powerful example of advocacy in action, and it may be tempting to think that all advocacy could follow this pattern. The evaluation of advocacy would then, exclusively, be a matter of asking partners whether the advocate had succeeded in getting their wishes implemented. But consider the following scenario:

Hassan

Hassan has dementia. He lives in a residential home near to his elderly sister, who visits regularly. Hassan has had a citizen advocate for six months. Now, social services propose that Hassan be moved to a nursing home further away, as this will offer more comprehensive care as his condition deteriorates. But his sister will not be able to visit him nearly so often. Hassan does not appear to understand the proposal to move him.

In this case there is no obvious 'answer' for the advocate to pursue; but this does not make the advocacy role any less vital. Hassan may need to be defended against a move that suits the services' needs rather than his own. The value of his relationship with his sister may need to be set against the clinical value of any proposed move. Hassan may well need support and reassurance through a time of considerable uncertainty. Any or all of these issues may require advocacy input. The role will be complex, and evaluating it difficult. Whereas explicit partner satisfaction was the *sole* criterion of the worth of advocacy in the previous example, here its role may well be negligible. Hassan may be able to say little or nothing about the advocate; he may not even *know* whether the advocate is doing well. The latter's role here would have to be judged in terms of factors such as their values and commitment, as well as the results these bring. Is the advocate doing their utmost to see the situation through Hassan's eyes? Do they have a real commitment to him as a person? How is this commitment shown in their actions? Far from being an impersonal instrument, here it is the advocate's personal qualities, and the quality of their relationship with Hassan, which are the defining facts of the partnership.

So in some advocacy situations, user feedback will be central to the evaluation of the support given. In other, equally important scenarios, it will not be possible to gain this feedback, and a broader spectrum of indicators will need to be used. These indicators are unlikely to be part of the Best Value approach, which (in line with the model in Figure 1) assumes that service organisations follow a single series of processes in order to deliver outcomes. This cannot be the case with advocacy.

The rationing agenda

In the section on the ambiguity of measurable outcomes, it was noted that ANNETTE, in anticipating the Best Value approach to advocacy, would be likely to give an advantage to schemes that could demonstrate a high 'throughput' of partners; in other words, schemes based on the casework model. This can be taken a stage further. May not a Best Value funder decide, not only that short-term advocacy is better than the citizen advocacy approach, because of its higher outputs, but that even short-term advocacy would be more efficient if it were time-limited? That is to say, every issue should be resolved, and every partnership ended, within a given timescale. Indeed, the authors are aware of at least one scheme which has to obtain its funder's permission if it wishes to work with an individual for more than a couple of months. From the Best Value perspective, this is a logical step; from the advocacy perspective, it is surely a fatal compromise of a scheme's independence. The two approaches are here irreconcilable.

The reasons for this conflict become clearer if we review some of the agendas that lie behind Best Value. It was stated earlier that Best Value grew out of the shift in industry and retail to a consistent and pervasive focus on the needs of the customer. But there is one important difference between retail consumers and the customers of public services. When someone buys an insurance policy (to continue our earlier example), they could be said to be an 'empowered' customer, since the insurer needs their premium as much as the customer needs the cover. Should the customer require two, four or a dozen policies, the insurer will be no less pleased with their custom – quite the opposite, in fact. In health and social services, however, the customers are not so empowered; our need for help or treatment is not matched by a corresponding need on the services' part to help us. In fact, given the limits to public finance, they often have an interest in rationing the services they provide. To some extent, this interest is counterbalanced by Patients Charters and other standards – but the rights contained in these documents are themselves defined by the rationing bodies: the providers and the government. The point is illustrated by the fact that even those who are generally confident and assertive can quickly feel powerless and humiliated when they receive poor healthcare, perhaps feeling the shock of being utterly dependent on clinicians who have no corresponding need, or apparent care, for them.

The reality of rationing means that in some respects, the Best Value approach undermines the 'customer first' ethos even as it apparently promotes it. In importing the Best Value approach into advocacy, there is a real danger of importing rationing, too. If this happens, one of the key tasks of advocacy – challenging the exclusion of individuals from services – is effectively neutered. Advocacy will have become another rationed, and rationing, service.

A middle way?

As things stand, then, the Best Value approach poses a number of threats to the practice of independent advocacy. Nor are these threats purely hypothetical; advocacy is already being influenced and, we have argued, its principles weakened by the demands of Best Value. The conflict which Wolfensberger and O'Brien portrayed between the service culture and the advocacy culture is as real as ever. The terms of the conflict, however, have changed and become more subtle; Best Value poses a threat to advocacy precisely because it seems to have assimilated some key advocacy values, such as 'putting the customer first'. These apparent values tend to blur a reality that is driven by 'outputs' and rationing, making it all too easy for advocacy to accommodate itself to issues it should be challenging.

But whatever the threats it poses, Best Value is here to stay: the advocacy movement cannot simply opt out of its demands for efficiency and demonstrable effectiveness, and still hope to attract public funding. It will in future be less and less possible to attract resources simply on the grounds that advocacy is 'worthwhile'. Is there a middle route between a wholesale capitulation to the service model which betrays the purpose of advocacy, and a retreat into purist isolationism which will see it wither on the vine as advocacy schemes continue to argue over what exactly 'purity' is? Such a middle way may be possible if the advocacy movement can produce its own account of what constitutes good advocacy; that is, if it can define advocacy outcomes, and the means used to deliver, monitor and evaluate them in terms which are credible to its users and to society at large, *and* which are distinct from those of the service culture. Achieving this would require much closer cooperation across the advocacy movement than exists at present.

This chapter began with attempts to establish a baseline for current advocacy provision. This task was complicated by the fact that, first, there are apparently insoluble arguments between different schools of advocacy which undermine the credibility of existing evaluation systems, and second that advocacy is in danger of being distorted rather than legitimised by the demands of Best Value. The chapter's conclusion has been that the advocacy movement must define itself in a way that is both distinctive and coherent in order to overcome these threats. This task of definition may best be begun by asking the fundamental question 'What is advocacy for?'

FOUR

What is advocacy for?

Ask the question 'What is advocacy?' and, as we have seen, one can quickly become mired in the arguments between different styles of advocacy. By asking what advocacy is *for*, we may be able to identify a range of outcomes that cuts across these different styles. This in turn may allow a refocusing of the advocacy movement around common endeavours. 'What is advocacy for?' seems a pertinent question, too, because advocacy (unlike, say, befriending) by definition aims at something beyond itself. Advocacy aims to bring about changes. If we wish to develop a strong advocacy culture, we must present these changes – or results – more clearly.

If advocacy means 'speaking up for another', it must involve integrity, conviction and wholeheartedness. A key test of this integrity will be whether the relationship with the other is in any way tainted by vested interests. But this will not be the only indicator; the quality of the advocate's rapport with their partner, and of the tasks they undertake on the partner's behalf, will also be important factors.

Advocacy schemes of all types have tried to codify these and other core values into principles which will regulate advocates' activity. Yet in reading almost any code of practice for advocates, one becomes aware of quite intense conflicting pressures within the role. The following, from a code of practice in the *Key ideas on independent advocacy* pack (Advocacy 2000, 2000)[1], is a good illustration of this:

> An advocate has the right to speak up on any issue ... which the advocate and their partner feel need attention.

> The advocate will not do anything on their partner's behalf without first making every effort to be sure that their partner wants them to. People with severe disabilities may not be able actually to speak and say what they want, but no matter how severe the disability people can usually find other ways of letting people know how they feel and what they want. (Advocacy 2000, 2000, section 6, p 16)[1]

There is a huge amount said, and still more implied within this relatively brief quote, which is worth analysing. It opens with a statement about the 'rights' of an advocate to represent another. These rights are considerable; they imply that the advocate speaks with authority on the partner's behalf and therefore should be heard. The image of the advocate here is of someone who is likely to have a bold and significant impact on the way services and society treat their partner.

The second statement places the advocate under an obligation that is at least as great as their 'rights' – to follow their partner's wishes at all times. Indeed, they are to make strenuous efforts to find out what these wishes are, however hard they are to identify. The image here is of the advocate as always cautious; any understanding they have of the partner may only be provisional. Is there a tension here between one principle which encourages advocates to speak up for partners because they have a special kind of commitment to (and even responsibility for) them, and another which requires the advocate to work in a highly self-critical way in order to achieve a dispassionate view of what the partner really wants? The first principle asserts that a strong identity between advocate and partner exists and is the basis of advocacy. The advocate represents the partner's wishes as though they were their own (O'Brien, 1987). The second principle is cautious, even sceptical about such identification; the advocate must continually check that their commitment is not obscuring the partner's wishes.

Advocacy principles are meant to tell advocates how to put key advocacy values into practice, but in this instance, two core principles appear to be in tension, if not in conflict. Neither can be discarded, since each is rooted in a value that lies at the heart of advocacy: on the one hand, the need for advocates to identify with those they speak up for, on the other, the need to respect the partner's autonomy. Instead of giving clear guidelines for action, the principles can in some real-life situations present us with a dilemma. The following story highlights this dilemma:

Jane

Alice has been Jane's citizen advocate for six months. Jane has a severe learning disability. Her face lights up when she sees Alice, and she likes showing Alice magazines and some of her treasured possessions. She seems happy at home.

Recently, other residents have complained about Jane's behaviour, and it is now proposed to move her to a more supported environment where she can be 'helped' with her behaviour. Service staff tell Alice they don't want to say too much too soon to Jane about the move "because she might get upset".

How should Alice proceed? Should she do everything she can to find out Jane's views, taking the risk that this will distress her without necessarily finding out her informed opinion? Should Alice simply challenge the decision to evict Jane from her home? Should she visit the proposed home herself, to see if it looks as though it may be right for Jane? She might do any of these, or pursue one of a number of other possibilities. What is clear, however, is that the principles of advocacy do not prescribe a single, simple course of action in this, nor in many other instances:

> Advocacy involves issues and problems which are not easily resolved, and which may not have a 'right answer'. People working in advocacy need to be aware of this and have strategies to deal with such problems. (Advocacy 2000, 2000, section 1, p 8)

A clear and coherent set of principles is essential to any advocacy undertaking; the responsibilities involved in speaking for another person in formal settings are far too great to be left to individual whim. But the preceding paragraphs suggest that no set of principles can satisfactorily dictate an advocate's course of action in all circumstances. There will be many situations where an advocate has to rely on their own judgement; and this judgement will be informed by the *kind* of relationship that exists between them and the advocacy partner. Why should this be? One answer may be that there are two conflicting currents or philosophies at work within advocacy, which need to be described more fully if we are to understand what advocacy is for.

There is a side to advocacy that has its roots in something other than principles and ideologies – in what one might term the 'moral drama' of everyday life. The following story illustrates this point:

Peter and Joan

Peter and Joan are working in their office. Erroll, their manager, comes in and starts to shout at Peter for delivering a piece of work late. Peter tries to defend himself, saying that Erroll has not made clear what he wanted, but his defence is met with a torrent of personal criticism. Erroll tells him he is a disappointment to the company, far less effective than person X in department Y, and the chief reason for recent poor performance.

At this point Joan speaks up. "I think you are being unfair. Peter asked you for more information on this two weeks ago and you never got back to him." Erroll is silenced and storms off. The crisis has been averted.

The power of such events is immediately apparent. Joan's speaking up on behalf of Peter has probably changed relationships within the office forever. Peter might have felt isolated by Erroll's tactics, but now feels he has an ally and is less likely to be picked on in future. Erroll may feel he has to rethink his whole managerial approach. Quite possibly, too, the event will have changed (if only a little) the way each character feels about themselves. Joan may have realised for the first time how much she dislikes power games. Peter may feel valued and therefore more confident in himself.

So, even in a simple advocacy scenario like this, many things can be happening, many changes taking place. But it is important to note, too, what is absent from this situation: Joan does not 'work out' how she should respond from a set of principles or ideas. What happened was spontaneous; that was why it was so powerful. Joan may subsequently rationalise the event, and decide that she was protecting Peter's rights as an employee – but the thought never entered her head at the time. Should Joan have sought Peter's permission before speaking up for him? The question simply never arose; it has no part in this drama.

If we follow this line of thinking, it is much easier to see why *relationships* are central to effective advocacy. It is relationships that generate drama; drama that changes relationships. Wolfensberger's genius in developing citizen advocacy lay in the fact that he put this sort of dynamic at the heart of the form; the citizen advocate's relationship to the partner should begin to transform their other less positive relationships. The citizen advocacy movement might find new energy and inspiration if it researched, developed and celebrated the idea of relationship (or partnership), and saw its principles as only the means to sustain relationships, rather than as an end in themselves.

Peer advocacy and self-advocacy, too, could be said to share in the idea of advocacy as 'drama'. It is important to say here that 'drama' does not refer to play-acting or over-the-top postures; it refers to all those real-life situations that can only be described in terms of actions and relationships, rather than ideas. No doubt it was an appreciation of the dramatic element in advocacy which led Wolfensberger and O'Brien to make the telling of partnership stories the primary means for recording achievements in citizen advocacy. Both peer and self-advocacy may be said to proceed likewise from a perception that any given advocacy 'problem' is likely to be a product of the much wider social and political situation in which the advocacy partner or self-advocate finds themselves. This situation is likely to consist of predominantly unequal or limiting relationships which result in a lack of opportunity, low expectations, and a sense of powerlessness. The peer advocate in speaking up for a user of mental health services is then not simply addressing a 'problem', but is also using their equality with the partner to demand a different type of service culture. If the peer advocate is successful, it will no longer be a case of the partner having to conform to the service before they are deemed to be 'better'; the service will have to value the partner *as they are*, and work *with* them in any treatment process. The self-advocate, similarly, is transforming a situation in which they have been seen as an essentially passive user of services into one where they are a key player in the drama.

Each of these three styles of advocacy, then, sees advocacy as capable of bringing about far-reaching changes in individuals' circumstances, status and self-perception. However, if drama can be transforming, it can also be clichéd, pretentious or boring. As we noted in the last chapter, the fact that a scheme employs a set of processes to bring about change is no guarantee that those changes are actually happening. Citizen and peer advocacy schemes need to find credible ways of ensuring and demonstrating the effectiveness of advocacy partnerships.

One or two more points need to be made about the dramatic element in advocacy. The first is to note the fundamental importance of what can happen when one human being identifies with another.

What has been said so far suggests that many advocacy partners find themselves in situations where negative factors continually reinforce one another. Being viewed as 'different' makes it much harder for people to be understood. Partners are therefore much more likely to be judged, and these judgements are likely to lead to overt or covert forms of exclusion or segregation. Long-term experience of this kind of negative cycle is likely to cause a great deal of pain. Where this devaluing cycle includes the trauma of abuse or other forms of harm, the pain will be so much the greater. In its extreme forms, this hurt is likely to destroy an individual's self-esteem, impair their relationships with others, and inhibit them from utilising such opportunities as do come their way. Simone Weil wrote that in affliction we lose the world (Wills, 1956, vol 1). To value someone who is otherwise devalued, to believe someone who is otherwise disbelieved, to stand by someone who is otherwise alone, may be a powerful means to help them 'find the world' again.

It is important to state at once that this is not an attempt to categorise advocacy as 'therapy', or users of advocacy as 'victims' or 'sufferers'. On the contrary, it is to suggest that *anyone* who is persistently exposed to negative, harmful or inappropriate environments may go through very deep experiences of hurt which cannot easily be communicated. The advocacy relationship offers the genuine commitment of another person who respects the partner's potential and encourages them to explore this in their own way and time. In doing so, advocacy can provide a non-judgemental arena in which the past can begin to be recovered, not as 'problem' or 'illness', but as human experience.

The advocate's identifying with their partner may touch on some deep human issues. But again, in recognising the power in an advocacy that arises spontaneously out of one person's genuine regard for another, we must recognise the possibility of failure here, too. To return to our original scenario: suppose Joan had simply stayed silent when Erroll was attacking Peter? She might well have felt scared, or unequal to the task. People are not always altruistic; they are rarely heroic; and it is a fact that some advocacy partnerships founder because the volunteer advocate cannot or will not stay the course. Equally, some partnerships fail because the advocate, no matter how committed or skilful, feels that they cannot get to know the partner, or understand their wishes. There may be 'failures' in advocacy which are the fault of no one; but this does not make redundant the question about whether or not individual partnerships and schemes are effective.

By considering advocacy as something that is first and foremost dramatic – a happening – rather than as something primarily to do with ideas, we can begin to understand why it is potentially so powerful, and why it may be difficult to codify in a series of rules. But this is only half the story. Consider another scenario:

Mary

Mary has a speech impediment. She has been asked to provide a witness statement in a civil court case. She feels strongly about the case, and wishes to present her statement 'live' in court, but fears she will not be understood if she reads it herself. She asks her longstanding neighbour, Jane, to read the statement for her. Jane agrees. She reads the statement as planned, Mary thanks her, and Jane then leaves the court while Mary remains to hear the outcome of the case.

This scenario is in many ways the opposite of the one described earlier in the chapter. There, there was a real threat to Peter's status as an employee; by identifying with him, Joan challenged the patterns and assumptions that gave rise to that threat. In this scenario, Mary faces an obstacle rather than a threat; she knows what she wants to say to the court, but needs help in saying it. Jane, in agreeing to read the statement, is *not* identifying with Mary: were she to read the statement as if the case affected her personally, the effect would be bizarre and inappropriate. Jane leaves court after reading the statement; although she is doubtless pleased to have helped Mary, her involvement does not give her any particular investment in the wider outcome.

Jane's advocacy for Mary is essentially non-dramatic; she is rather a proxy who has a simple role within a clearly defined situation. There is a similarity here with the account of advocacy given by Rachel Perkins, quoted in the last chapter. Jane provides the means for Mary to control the situation, whereas Joan speaks up *for* Peter because he is (temporarily) powerless. Both scenarios involve advocacy, but they highlight radically differing advocacy styles. Peter and Joan's story, which led on to a discussion of advocacy as drama, might be said to represent *personal* advocacy, whereas the Mary and Jane scenario epitomises *technical* advocacy. This distinction has some echoes of Wolfensberger's identification of 'expressive' and 'instrumental' advocacy roles. But whereas Wolfensberger saw these as complementary aspects of the citizen advocacy approach (on the one hand developing an empowering relationship with the partner, and on the other hand speaking up with or for them), personal and technical advocacy each represent complete, and in some ways contrasting, concepts of advocacy. The 'personal' advocate may well speak up for their partner, but their grounds for doing so will be very different from those of the technical advocate.

The personal advocate is likely to act out of empathy with, or concern for, the partner, born out of a personal commitment to them. Almost certainly, the advocate will have sought the partner's approval for their action, but the *idea* of raising an issue is quite likely to have come from the advocate themselves. In raising the issue, the advocate is likely to be moved by an unconceptualised wish for fairness, decency and respect for their partner. Technical advocacy aims at a particular outcome, and therefore generally presupposes a partner who is able to articulate this desired outcome. The advocate provides a series of skills, but the process is essentially controlled by the partner.

To some extent, the distinction between technical and personal advocacy is reflected in the differences between schemes which see themselves as undertaking casework, and those which define advocacy in terms of partnership. Schemes offering professional advocates would be a prime example of the former, citizen advocacy schemes of the latter. Schemes which provide volunteer advocates to support people through particular issues may combine elements of both approaches. By looking at the possible strengths and weaknesses of each model, one can begin to identify some key advocacy outcomes.

The casework approach

Strengths	Weaknesses
Advocates probably knowledgeable and skilled in dealing with service system	Casework is not generally preventive
The advocacy will more or less conform to a uniform standard	Requires clear direction from the user
Clear guidelines for user control of the advocacy process	May be identified as 'just another service' by users
'Professionalism' gains credibility with service workers	May not help those who want support, rather than choices
Relatively fast response times	Possibility of advocate 'burnout'

The partnership approach

Strengths

Solidarity – can transform perceptions of the partner

Allows partners' views to develop and change

Preventive effects

Escape from the service culture

Supports the person, not simply promoting their wishes

Weaknesses

Advocates' skill/expertise is variable

Standards may be harder to define

Varying credibility with the service system

Varying response times

If these suggestions are correct, it becomes apparent that neither approach can lay claim to the full range of advocacy outcomes. Casework may have little to offer someone who needs the support and commitment of another person in order to begin to recover self-esteem; partnership may not be relevant to someone who knows their own wishes but faces an acute problem with the authorities which will require expert help in order to be resolved. It is not possible to state that either the partnership or casework model is 'best'; this will depend on the situation of the advocacy partner.

This distinction between 'casework' and 'partnership' schemes, then, has some correspondence to the difference between technical and personal philosophies of advocacy. But the correspondence is not absolute. Citizen advocates may well find themselves embarked on a technical role, promoting their partner's explicit wishes in the face of indifference or obstruction. Caseworkers may find that they develop a strong personal commitment to some of the users of their scheme – perhaps to those who make repeated use of advocacy.

It is important that all advocacy schemes reflect on the relative emphasis that they place on these two contrasting philosophies. It is easy to fall into the belief that advocacy is 'all about choices' or 'all about loyalty' but each view has its pitfalls. Advocacy schemes need to be aware that principles which serve some of their partners well may be less helpful to others; they should guard against too narrow a definition of 'what advocacy is for'. As we saw in the last chapter, the Best Value funding regime favours the technical/casework approach;

advocacy that aims at support, prevention and personal development is threatened. This is not just a threat to the future of citizen advocacy, although it is here that the threat is most apparent; it is a threat to advocacy as a whole. For even within casework advocacy, as we have seen, the personal rapport between advocate and partner may be essential to the success of the role. If this personal element does not continue to be highlighted across all schemes, if people are only cases to be processed, advocacy loses its rationale. People who are not supported, protected from abuse or sustained in their development of self-esteem may, as we have seen, become people who are too disempowered or despairing to voice their wishes or direct their lives. In this sense, the more tangible processes of technical advocacy depend on the deeper objectives of personal advocacy being met. The advocacy movement must remain alert enough to include both philosophies, and the funding environment should permit each to flourish.

The personal and technical philosophies mark out two distinct, but interdependent approaches to the question 'What is advocacy for?' Studying them has helped to begin to shape a list of advocacy outcomes: for example, prevention and user control (or choice) were mentioned in the analyses of casework and partnership. It may now be helpful to have a suggested inventory of outcomes. These will, of necessity, have to be fairly generalised; nonetheless they should provide some indication of what it is that makes advocacy distinctive. The following list of advocacy outcomes is a 'first try' that will hopefully form the basis for further discussion and refinement by others within the advocacy movement:

- Choice
- Access
- Justice
- Social development
- Support
- Empowerment
- Prevention.

Each of these outcomes needs describing more fully.

Choice

To choose is to make a difference; it is also to *make oneself* different. The myriad choices that most people make in the course of a day influence and change the environment around them in more or less subtle ways. But a person's choices, precisely because they are individual to them, play a key role in shaping other people's perceptions of who that person is, too. We may warm or cool towards people according to the type of music they choose to play, or clothes they choose to wear, or behaviour they choose to exhibit. To choose is to begin to act as a definite person, rather than merely existing as furniture in the lives of others.

Many people seek advocacy support because their choices are obstructed. A disabled person wishing to live at home may be told that their support needs are 'too expensive' and that they must accept residential care instead. A looked after young person may feel that their foster carers are stifling their development with petty 'house rules'. An older person who wishes to continue looking after their own money may feel threatened by a friend or relative who seeks receivership. In all of these instances, where the partner's choice is disregarded, their influence over key elements of their personal environment is removed. Nor is there simply an external loss; people who have had what are otherwise basic rights taken away from them are likely to feel hurt, angry or worthless – or a mixture of the three. In taking up issues of choice, advocates may not simply be influencing what happens; they may be challenging long-held assumptions on the part of society, or helping individuals to maintain or recover a sense of self-worth.

The greatest strength of technical advocacy is in promoting the choices of partners who would otherwise not be heard. The following story illustrates how effective this can be:

Andrew

Andrew lives with foster-carers. He would like to join a youth club trip to Paris, but both his carers and his social worker oppose the idea.

Andrew's advocate, Jim, contacts the social worker and repeats Andrew's wish.

"There are things you don't know about Andrew which might change your view", says the social worker.

"It's not my view, it's Andrew's wish", replies Jim. "And I don't really want to know any more about him than he is prepared to tell me himself."

"You saw his behaviour yesterday; no one could travel in that state."

"He was upset because you *told* him he couldn't go. Anyway, why does he have to earn the right to go; none of the other kids do. He'd accept the same rules as them; anyone misbehaving is sent home."

"Well ... he has no idea about money", the social worker continues.

"He's had no chance to learn with his current carers. Besides, I have spoken to the youth leader and he would help Andrew to manage."

"Even if I agree, his carers won't...."

"I'm happy to talk to them", says Jim.

The anecdote illustrates some of the many obstacles that can be put in the way of choice: professional 'secrets', character judgements, the partner's supposed 'inability', and the appeal to 'powerful others'. It also shows how an advocate who is focused on the partner's choice can use information, argument and tenacity to overcome these obstacles. From first to last, the partner's wish is kept centre stage.

On the other hand, people who have experienced institutionalisation or other forms of chronic disadvantage, as we have seen, seem sometimes to lose the ability to choose altogether. What we have termed 'personal advocacy' can play a significant part in helping people to recover the sense of confidence and self-worth which are the foundations on which choice is built, as Ernie's story illustrates:

> When I do see him, just to see his face, how happy he is to see me ... that alone ... you can't buy that! I am there for him. He can't speak, and we're trying to work on developing signs. I think from years ago he just stopped talking. He was probably left to his own devices and didn't find the need to talk. (Williams, 1998, p 45)

In Ernie's case, identifying his choices is a very long-term affair. But the citizen advocate remains motivated to help Ernie, sensing and respecting his potential. At present, Ernie does not express his personality through choices; his personality is only expressed through free and creative relationships such as that which he has established with his advocate. In this scenario, only a personal advocacy approach can be effective.

Perhaps the most fundamental of all choices is that between 'yes' and 'no'. 'No' in particular can be described as the first step in choosing because it marks a refusal of others' version of the world, of their plans or wishes. Many of those who choose the support of an advocate do so because they are involved in an unequal struggle, often with the service system. There may be huge, unspoken, pressures to go along with whatever doctors, social workers or housing officers decree. Because advocates are outside of the service relationship, and not expected to be 'grateful', they can express their partners' disagreement or refusal confidently and consistently.

It is often remarked that the simple introduction of an advocate to an individual can have a significant, positive effect on the way services treat them. Professionals may become more respectful of the partner, more likely to offer choices than ready-made solutions. One reason for this is that the very presence of an advocate raises the possibility of an effective 'no' to the system. This kind of effect is extremely difficult to monitor or record; perhaps advocates could note whether their partners are indeed offered choices once the advocate is involved, or whether the solutions offered are demonstrably needs-led rather than service-led.

Another key area of choice concerns an individual's right to take risks, even to make mistakes. In the past it was the institutional nature of services which prevented service users from doing anything that departed from the 'norms' set by the regime. Some of these restrictions have disappeared with the advent of independent living and care in the community, but the culture of risk management threatens to create further barriers. The pressures of risk management are perhaps most acute in relation to child protection. Many disabled and learning disabled parents have faced the prospect of having their children removed by the local authority on the grounds that their disability and/or living circumstances pose a risk to the children's well-being. The child protection system focuses absolutely on the interests of the child; it is therefore essential that parents have recourse to advocacy (if they want it) so that their wish to bring up their children is given a full and fair hearing, and all feasible avenues for realising this wish are explored. In many such instances, there will be a need for strong technical advocacy, negotiating skilfully with a range of agencies in pursuit of the parents' wishes. There may also be a need for personal advocacy, supporting parents through a bleak and stressful time, whatever the outcome.

Advocates help people to identify and express choices. More than this, they seek to make their partners' choices effective, even decisive. The styles of advocacy used to pursue these ends will vary, as will the means of monitoring their success; nonetheless choice remains a key advocacy outcome.

Access

The choices available to a person at any given time tend only to be as good as their general life situation. Someone living in a hostel for disabled people may have a considerable degree of choice and control within that environment, and yet still lack both opportunity and acceptance within the wider community. An individual living in this situation may simply not know of the ways in which they could make their life better. Advocacy plays a significant role, therefore, not only in representing people's choices, but also in providing the information on which those choices can be based.

Both technical and personal advocacy have a role to play in creating access though, here as elsewhere, the respective approaches are different to the point of seeming contradictory. Perhaps the differences are best illustrated through two scenarios.

Access: technical advocacy

Mark is a sessional worker with a professional advocacy scheme. Rashid is a disabled man who lives in his own flat. Rashid has asked to see Mark because he feels he is getting no support in developing his quality of life. Mark asks Rashid about his current situation, and how he would like this to develop. Would he like to work? How would he like his social life to develop? And so on. He notes Rashid's answers and after the meeting researches local services and opportunities which he thinks would most closely meet Rashid's needs. He meets Rashid again to find out which of these avenues he wishes to pursue. Finally, he agrees with Rashid how he should put a case to the local authority for the additional support hours Rashid will need to realise his wishes.

In this scenario, Mark plays a vital role in bringing information to Rashid, which enables him to make concrete plans for developing his life. But Mark is careful throughout not to impose his own views as to how Rashid should act, nor to seek to influence his choices. The whole point of the advocacy exercise is that it should be owned by Rashid. It would perhaps be wrong to talk of an advocacy 'partnership' in this instance; Mark's role is more that of facilitator than peer or colleague.

Access: personal advocacy

Mary is undergoing the latest in a long series of hospitalisations for mental health problems. She is quiet and withdrawn, refusing to attend occupational therapy. Some staff feel she is being deliberately uncooperative.

The citizen advocacy coordinator, Jane, has heard of Mary via a relative, and asks if she can visit her. Her initial questions to Mary are met with silence. Then Jane notices that Mary has a tape of an opera beside her bed. She tells Mary: "I know a woman who loves opera. I think she would like to meet you. Could I bring her in sometime?". Mary nods slightly.

Over the following weeks, Anna becomes Mary's citizen advocate. They listen to music together, and Mary makes the occasional comment. When Mary's section is due for renewal, Anna asks if she agrees to this. Mary shakes her head, but does not answer Anna's follow-up questions about what she, Mary, would like to happen in the future.

Jane and Anna's approach with Mary is almost the opposite of Mark's with Rashid. Whereas in the first scenario it was important that Mark kept his personality out of the advocacy process, here Anna's character is essential to its success. In the second scenario, advocacy is precisely about building a partnership; it is Mary's personal relationship with Anna, rather than any information that Anna brings which will – hopefully – create a bridge to a better life for her. The advocacy tasks that Anna performs for Mary (representing her at tribunal and so on) will be informed by this relationship, as much as by any overt choices Mary has made.

The two scenarios represent extremes of technical and personal advocacy. In helping partners to access greater opportunity, advocacy schemes will be supporting people who may at different times need *both* personal and technical advocacy support. The challenge for schemes is first, to be aware of these different (perhaps conflicting) needs, and then to utilise their resources to meet them. Within a citizen advocacy scheme, this will mean ensuring that the advocate really is the 'right' person for their partner. How is this decision made? Within a casework scheme it will mean ensuring that advocates are skilled enough to offer different styles of support to different people.

Justice

A simple, working definition of justice would be: the full realisation of a person's rights, and redress for any wrongs inflicted on them. The quest for justice lies at the heart of advocacy; it is the recognition that injustice can and often does occur that has brought organised advocacy into being; it was the uncovering of abuse within long-stay hospitals which led to the creation of the first citizen advocacy schemes in the UK.

If there is a popular image of advocacy, it is probably of an advocate pleading a partner's cause within a meeting, tribunal or case conference, convincing powerful individuals or organisations that they should value the partner more highly, or treat them with greater fairness.

Angie

Angie is in her mid-20s, and has mild learning and physical disabilities. She wished to attend her local college to undertake a BTEC course. To do this she would need the provision of transport and personal support while at college. Angie's advocate, Irene, was brought in to help her negotiate this provision. Both the college and the local authority made offers of support which were not enough. When Irene objected and asked how these offers had been calculated (there appeared to have been no assessment of Angie's needs) it was implied that Angie should be grateful for whatever she was given. Irene researched the legislation covering social services provision, and Further Education Funding Council guidelines on the inclusion of disabled students. When she relayed the results of her enquiries to the college and local authority, much better levels of help were promised, and Angie was able to start her course.

This popular image stresses the more technical aspect of advocacy, portraying the advocate as a skilled negotiator upholding the partner's wishes in a difficult or even hostile environment.

Angie's story, like that of Andrew earlier in the chapter, highlights some of the key ingredients which make technical advocacy successful:

- *Assertiveness.* Irene and Angie were not bought off by the suggestion they should be grateful for what was offered.
- *Knowledge.* Being able to locate the relevant legislation and guidelines helped Irene to put together a convincing argument.
- *Negotiating skills.* Irene was able to show that the authorities' initial position was flawed, since no proper assessment had been made of Angie's needs.

Any advocacy scheme can and should ask itself how it helps its advocates to develop these faculties.

Though technical advocacy skills will be to the fore in seeking justice for partners, personal advocacy also has an important part to play. As noted before, people who have experienced long-term injustices (abuse, institutionalisation) will be far less likely to find their way to an advocacy scheme, or to express clear-cut choices. There is a vital role for advocacy schemes which can identify deeply disadvantaged groups and individuals and create long-term advocacy partnerships which will gradually raise partners' expectations and the standards of their services.

Speaking up for justice can be highly contentious; an advocate who speaks up passionately for their partner's cause may encounter equally forceful opposition. It is far from unknown for advocates who have challenged the status quo to have their integrity or competence questioned. Such conflicts become even more complex if the organisation being challenged (for example, a local authority) is also the scheme's main funder. There will quite possibly be pressure on the scheme (spoken or unspoken) to tone down its advocacy or face withdrawal of funding. While the present, unsatisfactory arrangements for advocacy funding persist, a key part of any evaluation must surely focus on how a scheme challenges its funder, and how these challenges affect both individual partners, and the provision of advocacy in general.

Social development

Advocacy evaluation systems to date have failed to highlight advocacy's impact on the development of society at large. This is puzzling, given that advocacy, if it has any meaning at all, consists of a series of 'live encounters' with issues of rights, disadvantage and justice. In laying bare the unfairness or impracticality of rules and regulations, advocates are demonstrating the need for these to be changed. As David Brandon records (Brandon, 1995), MIND's advocacy in the early 1980s was geared to just these sorts of outcomes.

Personal advocacy plays a part here, too. Citizen advocacy schemes have always held that by valuing otherwise marginalised people, advocacy demonstrates the possibility of a more inclusive, less prejudiced society. Citizen advocacy partnerships make the point that not every human need can (or indeed, should) be met by the creation of a specialist 'service'. Personal advocacy makes the case for, and helps to build, a less compartmentalised society.

There is no easy measure of a scheme's social impact, but the following indicators may help to outline this. A scheme might ask itself whether its advocacy has:

- helped create, or widen access to, innovative, needs-led services
- challenged and/or altered organisational procedures
- attracted positive media coverage
- helped people to gain independence as members of the community
- challenged discrimination.

Support

In looking at the differences between technical and personal advocacy, we suggested that while technical advocacy aims primarily at the realisation of the partner's stated choices, personal advocacy can be a source of long-term development and empowerment for people whose wishes are, for whatever reason, unclear. An advocate whose role is not time-limited, and who is there not as part of a service intervention, but out of loyalty to their partner, can help that person through the states of anger, despair and disorientation that may result from trauma or ongoing hardship, to the point where they begin to 'find the world' again.

Miriam

Social services initiated proceedings to have Miriam's child taken into care, and then offered for adoption. Dee acted as Miriam's advocate throughout this process, helping her to liaise with her solicitor, obtaining better support from social services, and finally going with her to the court hearing. Miriam lost her case, and her child was adopted.

Dee continued to support Miriam through the difficult months that followed. Shocked by her loss, Miriam first had thoughts of having another child, then of harming herself. Dee's loyalty and willingness to listen helped her get through this period. Slowly, Miriam began to plan for a more positive future.

It is sometimes argued that this sort of supportive role is 'just befriending', and not really advocacy at all. Certainly, had Dee been offering purely technical advocacy, her role would have ended with the loss of the court case. This, however, would have left Miriam in crisis. Instead, Dee was able to build on the relationship she had developed with Miriam to offer her empathy and encouragement. What had been, for Miriam, an entirely negative and depersonalising encounter with the service culture began to be transformed into a manageable, if profoundly sad, personal experience. Dee's role was not 'just befriending' because where befriending is essentially *aimless*, Dee had a clear goal: to help Miriam through a period of turmoil, to the point where she could begin to make choices informed by hope rather than anger.

If the advocacy movement gives up its role in supporting these sorts of personal outcomes, it will lose much of its soul. There is pressure for it to do just this. As we have seen, funders increasingly are opting to support advocacy that is time-limited and task-driven. The government's sponsorship of Patient Advocacy and Liaison Service (PALS) within the NHS looks set to continue this trend; the confusion of advocacy and liaison in the scheme's title suggests that it may be as much about improving the system (and thereby reducing litigation?) as about supporting the patient. Of course, advocacy can help service systems to work better, but this is not its rationale; it exists to promote the value, interests and wishes of the individual.

Empowerment

Empowerment, like advocacy itself, is widely acclaimed but difficult to measure. This is not to deny that it is a genuine outcome of good advocacy; and it is worth reflecting on some of the ways in which advocacy promotes empowerment.

If empowerment is the growth of an individual's ability to direct their own actions and influence their environment, then there are strong links between empowerment and choice. If advocacy helps someone to make a choice that was previously denied them (for example, to change their accommodation), that person may in future feel much more confident in voicing similar choices – perhaps now without an advocate's support. Empowerment may therefore be a long-term benefit accompanying more immediate advocacy outcomes.

Individual empowerment may be particularly connected with the development of self-advocacy skills. The growth of the self-advocacy movement in the past decade has highlighted how effective people with learning disabilities or mental health problems can be as negotiators, organisers and campaigners. Mindful of these achievements, advocacy schemes have often included a reminder of the importance of self-advocacy in their codes of practice:

> An independent professional advocate aims to support people to represent their own interests where possible and very much as a preference to acting on their behalf. (Advocacy 2000, 2000, Section 1, p 12)

Nonetheless, the issue of empowerment sometimes appears to be a source of confusion or conflict between advocacy and self-advocacy groups. A similar extract from Atkinson (1999) highlights this:

> Advocacy takes many forms but is essentially about speaking up – wherever possible for oneself (self advocacy), but sometimes with others (group or collective advocacy) and, where necessary, through others. (Atkinson, 1999, p 5)

This passage can be read in two ways. If it is stating that advocacy should begin with an affirmation of people's abilities, rather than assumptions about their disabilities, this is quite true. One sometimes hears it said that 'every service user should have an advocate'. Well-meant though such statements are, they reinforce the negative perception of service users as needy recipients. No one should have an advocate who does not want or need one. However, the Atkinson quote can also be read as suggesting that any advocacy which is not self-advocacy is by its very nature second best. This is misleading. All of us benefit from others' help at times; and throughout the course of our life it is our relationships with others which tend to be the most significant source of our personal development. To imply that those who receive support from an advocate are doing something less valid than those who advocate for themselves would be both untrue and divisive. The empowerment that comes through successful advocacy partnerships should be celebrated in the same way, and for the same reasons, as self-advocacy.

Prevention

By its nature, the prevention of harm, abuse or injustice is perhaps the most difficult of all advocacy outcomes to measure. How does one record something which has *not* happened *and* demonstrate that its non-happening was the result of advocacy? Yet, time and again, schemes find circumstantial evidence that the very presence of an advocate seems to have led to an improvement in their partner's circumstances.

Perhaps it is the confidential nature of the relationship between advocate and partner which is the key here. When an organisation believes that it 'knows all about' an individual, a terrible determinism can creep into its dealings with that person. One sees this clearly in the power of the 'labels' that services apply to people – labels such as 'schizophrenic', 'challenging' and so on; the person becomes indistinguishable from their 'problem'. It probably happens in less obvious ways too: the person with profound learning disabilities who is only ever seen in the routine settings of hostel, minibus and day centre may be perceived as little more than the sum of the services they receive. If such a person has an advocate, whose dealings with them are confidential, there is at once something 'not known' about that person, a distance which commands respect. They are seen as a person with interests; interests which do not necessarily coincide with those of their service provider.

Despite the difficulties in measuring these sorts of effects, advocacy schemes may be able to develop indicators which at least show that they are tackling issues of prevention seriously and systematically. A scheme might record:

- How it identifies people 'at risk' – such people are unlikely to find their own way to a scheme.
- What proactive steps does it take to find them, and what criteria does it use to support this process?
- How many people does it identify through this process?
- What skills do advocates offer to vulnerable people, and how does the scheme support and develop these skills?
- How do advocates help people to avoid risk? For example, by
  - informing people of their rights
  - arranging legal support for partners
  - representing formal complaints
  - helping to report abuse
  - preventing financial exploitation
  - helping to foster high expectations
  - actively monitoring services.

Doubtless this list could be developed further. Schemes that can offer a range of personal and technical advocacy approaches can play a key role in protecting people from injustice and maltreatment.

This chapter has attempted to provide some answers to the question 'What is advocacy for?' It has suggested that there are two key sources of advocacy. The first is bound up with the 'drama' of ordinary human relationships, one person supporting and speaking up for another out of a concern that does not require a highly developed conceptual base. This we termed 'personal advocacy'. The second source is in the much more specialised process of one person carrying through another's wishes in the face of physical or bureaucratic obstruction. This was termed 'technical advocacy'. Though these two sources are contrasting, and may at times appear to conflict, neither can do without the other. Good advocacy practice in part consists of managing the tension between the two; knowing when personal advocacy is needed, and when a more technical approach is required. We then proposed a series of general outcomes which might describe the overall results of effective advocacy.

If this, or a similar series of outcomes was acceptable to the advocacy movement as a whole, it might form one foundation of what Atkinson (1999) described as an 'advocacy culture'. How this might further be developed, and what its implications could be, are the subject of the next chapter.

Note

[1] The *Key ideas* pack draws on material from a range of schemes, but the views represented in it are not necessarily those of Advocacy 2000.

FIVE

Developing an advocacy culture

The last chapter proposed a series of general advocacy outcomes as the foundation for what Atkinson (1999) termed an 'advocacy culture'. The present chapter will look at the ways in which this advocacy culture can be developed. There are three key reasons for seeking to do this:

The inadequacy of the service model. Chapter Three suggested that many aspects of Best Value culture, such as its reliance on quantitative indicators of success, are not only inappropriate for, but damaging to, the implementation of good advocacy. In Chapter Four we saw that the service model is particularly ill-suited to describing the practice of personal advocacy – advocacy which offers both support and protection to the individual, and helps them to develop choices and opportunities over a period of time. Hence there is a need for a credible alternative model for advocacy practice.

Independence. Chapter Two highlighted the many ways in which the independence of advocates and advocacy schemes may be threatened or compromised. These threats will always exist as long as advocacy has to operate in an environment the parameters of which are set, not by the principles of advocacy, but by the requirements of service organisations. If the *practice* of advocacy can be established as distinctive and valuable in its own right, it will be far more difficult for non-advocacy interests to influence, manipulate or control it.

Funding. Insecurity of funding is a further significant threat to advocacy schemes. Most of the schemes spoken to in the course of preparing this work cited it as a problem. An advocacy movement that is clear about its identity will be much better placed to lobby for non-compromising and reliable sources of funding.

One way forward may be to develop a general model for what happens within an advocacy scheme. Like the outcomes proposed in the last chapter, this model would need to be broad enough to cover the many different types of advocacy scheme, but still sufficiently distinctive to *add something* to the understanding of advocacy. Such a model could help to 'ring-fence' advocacy against further encroachment by the service culture. It could also give helpful pointers for the development of new schemes, and the strengthening of existing ones.

Aside from these pragmatic motives for trying to develop an advocacy model, there is another, much simpler one: advocacy *is* unique. Few other spheres of social activity can claim such a rich combination of user involvement and personal commitment, or such a wide range of outcomes. Perhaps the high levels of motivation encountered among advocates and advocacy workers stem from the fact that this remarkable array of resources is entirely focused on the infinite possibilities of the individual. A strong advocacy scheme is a cultural entity in its own right. Seen from this perspective, it can be said that advocacy improves people's access to, and experience of services, not because it is a kind of 'super-service', but because it has a wholly different kind of relationship with its users. Advocacy centres on a unique type of relationship; and it is this relationship which establishes the credibility and legitimacy of the advocate's endeavours. This relationship reflects not only the advocate's encounter with the partner, but the whole ethos of the advocacy scheme. This benign view of advocacy can only be sustained, however, if within the advocacy culture there are installed valid means for differentiating good and bad advocacy. Distinctiveness cannot mean non-accountability; in proposing a new model for advocacy processes we shall need to return to the question of advocacy evaluation.

The model proposed is a model of the work of advocacy schemes, rather than of individual advocacy partnerships. Whereas the service model given in Chapter Three is built around the idea of a simple intervention, or set of interventions, which is repeated with each service user, no such simple, linear approach will truly portray the diverse processes at work within advocacy partnerships. The outcomes of advocacy are too varied to allow such a prescriptive approach. Instead, we can try to develop a framework for advocacy schemes, which will build on elements that many if not most schemes will already take for granted, but which presents these elements in a way which clarifies what is already happening, *and* encourages the perception of common endeavours across the advocacy movement.

Figure 2: A model for advocacy schemes

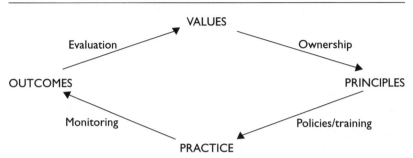

Three main considerations underpin the model's relevance to the advocacy movement:

- It places values at the heart of the advocacy enterprise. More will be said of this shortly.
- Rather than focus exclusively on issues of ownership and principles (as has often been the case in debates within the advocacy movement) or on practice and outcomes (as tends to be the case with the Best Value philosophy) the model seeks to present a broader, more inclusive context for advocacy development.
- Funding and funders are deliberately excluded from the process model, in order to uphold the independence of advocacy. Funding needs to be considered separately, and this is done towards the end of this chapter.

Each aspect of the model now needs to be described in more detail.

Values

Advocacy is values-driven: it begins with a vision, not with a series of prescribed tasks. This vision is not uniform across the advocacy movement, but within each scheme there is likely to be a set of strongly held social ideals which will govern both *what* the scheme is trying to achieve, and *how* it goes about this. We noted in Chapter Three that there tends to be an overlap of aims and principles in advocacy. This is borne out by the outcomes (or realised aims) listed at the end of Chapter Four; at least three of these – choice, justice and empowerment – are core values that will also determine *how* the scheme is run. Whereas, in business, values are subordinate to outcomes, in advocacy, there is parity between the two.

The values-driven nature of advocacy is inescapable. For we have seen that attempts to 'trim down' advocacy, to make it fit better with the service culture and Best Value ideals, lead to undue emphasis on 'technical' advocacy, and the neglect of significant areas of personal disadvantage. This threatens to turn advocacy partners into 'consumers'. But if the idealistic nature of advocacy makes each advocacy partnership potentially pioneering and exemplary, it also carries the threat of complacency and tokenism. Just as we saw in Chapter Three that the creation of a 'principled' advocacy partnership in no way ensures the success of that partnership, so it must be stated that the adoption of a powerful set of values does not in itself demonstrate that an advocacy scheme is worthwhile. The other stages of the model will be needed to establish this. The model is, among other things, a testing ground for the validity of advocacy values.

Ownership

It is ownership of core values by a committed group – often a steering group or management committee – which begins to turn aspirations into realities. In recent years, the ownership of service organisations has been a major issue for the disability movement. The notion that disabled people must be looked after by non-disabled people who 'know best' has thankfully been eroded over the past two decades, to the point where most major grant-giving bodies will now only make awards to organisations which can demonstrate significant levels of user-involvement in their management. Advocacy has not been unaffected by this process. As Atkinson (1999) attests, there has been some suspicion of the citizen advocacy form among disability groups, who view it as perpetuating a stereotype of dependency. Both peer and self-advocacy, in their different ways, seek to ensure that advocacy is controlled by disabled people, and does not become another form of exploitation.

Those involved with citizen advocacy would, however, oppose the idea that it undermines or marginalises disabled people, founded as it is on ideas of common citizenship and common humanity. It is worth considering here this argument about control and ownership in advocacy in a little more depth, since it highlights some of the suspicions and misunderstandings that currently weaken the advocacy movement. In the first instance, it is important to distinguish the *ownership* of a scheme (who manages it) from the control of its advocacy processes (who instructs the advocate). Those who manage or 'own' an advocacy scheme are not there to bestow expertise on clients. In advocacy, the client or partner *is* the expert, in the sense that it is their values, priorities, needs and experiences which form the bedrock of any given advocacy scenario. One might say that the advocate's role is to make the partner's expertise visible and effective.

Sometimes this is a relatively straightforward process, as is the case with technical advocacy scenarios. Here, as we have seen, the advocate is directed by the user's explicit wishes and conveys these to others. But in many other situations, the partner does not 'instruct' the advocate in this obvious manner. An individual who is isolated or institutionalised may have little concept of rights or choices, and it may take weeks or months to develop a sufficient rapport with them for their true wishes and interests to become apparent. Yet this personal advocacy approach is still founded on the belief that the partner has an expertise – a unique and irreplaceable perspective – which needs to be fostered and respected. Thus here, too, it is the partner's expertise which directs the partnership.

So issues of ownership and control in advocacy are much more complex than they may at first appear. Managing an advocacy scheme is not about controlling the advocacy it provides, but about making advocacy available to individuals in the way that will be most empowering to them. It is to the credit of the citizen advocacy form that it has always enshrined this principle. CAPE speaks approvingly, for example, of

> Advocates disagreeing with advocacy office staff about the nature of a [partner's] need, or the means to meet that need. (O'Brein and Wolfensberger, 1979, p 5)

The charge that citizen advocacy institutionally promotes dependency cannot therefore be maintained; the partner's needs should clearly come before those of the scheme in a successful partnership. Of course, there may be some individual citizen advocates who misrepresent their partners, and it is important that schemes challenge these advocates; but then failure is a possibility in *all* forms of advocacy.

There is probably no single ideal standard for the make-up of a steering group or management committee; needs will differ from one scheme, and one place, to another. What can be said is that the experiences of users of services are in one way or another fundamental to the development of schemes. It is these experiences – of injustice, of empowerment, of exclusion overcome – which bring a scheme's core values to life. Such experiences also highlight areas of advocacy need. There are at least three ways in which schemes can be informed by these experiences:

- by including service users and representatives of other disadvantaged groups in the scheme's management, staff, and pool of advocates
- by liaising with representative groups
- by reflecting on the experiences of the scheme's own advocacy partners.

The ownership of schemes needs to be effective as well as representative, however. Tasks such as management, recruitment, monitoring and fundraising all require skill. While a scheme may not include all desirable skills among its steering group at the outset, it should surely work towards this. Indeed, there seems no reason why evaluations of advocacy schemes should not look both at who is represented on the steering group, and at the skills they possess. There needs to be a balance between the two.

The issue of ownership also has a bearing on the comments made in Chapter Two about the structural independence of schemes. There it was noted that while some schemes are constituted in their own right, others operate under the umbrella of a Council for Voluntary Service (CVS) or are directly managed by national voluntary organisations. A commitment to building a distinctive advocacy culture does not appear to sit easily with the ownership of advocacy schemes by non-advocacy organisations. Of course, there are exceptions to this generalisation: where a group of people decides to start an advocacy scheme, they may initially seek developmental and administrative support from a CVS or voluntary organisation, until the project is established. So there can be no absolute rule for how advocacy schemes are managed. What can be said quite categorically, however, is this: to the extent that the ownership and management of a scheme reflect non-advocacy agendas, so far will the independence and quality of its advocacy be compromised. Sometimes these conflicts of interest will be blatant, as where an organisation runs an advocacy scheme and a rehabilitation hostel for mental health users in the same area, but they may also be subtle. Advocacy carries a good deal of credibility, and the 'contract culture' raises the prospect of what are essentially large service organisations 'buying in' to advocacy in order to enhance their 'brand value'. Corporate culture and advocacy culture should be kept well apart.

Who owns PALS?

The issue of ownership is especially pertinent to the government's ideas for a new Patient Advocacy Liaison Service (PALS) for the NHS. The government intends to abolish Community Health Councils (CHCs) which have hitherto exercised a watchdog function in the NHS, and instead require that all general hospitals should accommodate a patient advocate, based in the hospital's reception area and therefore accessible to all. The advocate will be employed by the hospital trust.

It is encouraging to see advocacy, hitherto very much at the margin of national and local government thinking, now suddenly thrust to the top of the policy agenda in relation to the NHS. The fairly large worm in this otherwise promising bud is, of course, the fact that the advocacy will be owned by the very hospital trusts it exists to monitor and to challenge. This will create considerable conflicts of interests. It will be a remarkable advocate who can help a patient expose facts that are damaging to the trust's public image; and it will be a remarkable trust that does not seek to tone down an advocate's potential impact through control, manipulation or undermining. The compromised ownership of PALS may have more direct impacts on the quality of the advocacy they give, too. There is likely to be considerable demand on PALS; advocates are therefore likely to find themselves under a pressure of numbers scarcely less than that confronting doctors and nurses. In this situation, will there not be a tendency for the advocacy to be highly technical, concentrating on the processes of hospitalisation ('when will surgery happen?' and so on) at the expense, for example, of the patient who is too upset or confused to challenge their consultant's recommendations? PALS may challenge some of the deficiencies of hospital systems; it is not clear that they will resolve the very deep sense of disempowerment often felt by patients within those systems.

It is not hard to see why the government should have chosen this 'in-house' model for PALS. The NHS is after all not just a provider of health care. It is also a very large political football. In independent hands, NHS advocacy might provide a rich mine of more or less sensational material for political opponents anxious to make political capital, and for journalists. With regard to the NHS, it is perhaps hard to say just who *is* independent. Nonetheless, the high profile adoption of the PALS model hinders rather than helps the development of an advocacy culture, since it gives a tacit nod to other large service organisations which would be only too happy to create 'in-house' advocacy for their users, and to dispense with the rigours of independent scrutiny.

Principles

Returning to the model, 'principles' will dictate the kind of tasks an advocacy scheme will undertake, and how it will undertake them. The principles will reflect the scheme's overall values, but will refer directly to advocacy rather than to the wider social context. Principles vary considerably from scheme to scheme, but the 'Key ideas' identified by Advocacy 2000 after widespread consultation with schemes in Scotland provide a valuable summary:

> There are lots of ways advocacy projects can be organised but good ones will have these important ideas in common:
> * Independence
> * Inclusion and respect
> * Empowerment
> * Loyalty
> * Safeguarding quality
> * Advocacy dilemmas. (Advocacy 2000, 2000, section 1, p 8)

Again, there is a degree of overlap between principles and outcomes (empowerment, inclusion); this as we have seen reflects the fact that advocacy is about convictions. The 'Key ideas' form a potentially useful benchmark for authentic advocacy, but they are abstract. How should schemes determine the kind, or kinds, of advocacy they will practise? Hitherto, this decision has tended either to be taken by schemes themselves, on the grounds that one form of advocacy (citizen, professional casework and so on) is 'the best', or else by funders who feel that a particular form (usually casework) represents Best Value. Can this process be refined, so that it incorporates not only conviction, but also an attempt to analyse need?

The analysis of advocacy as incorporating both technical and personal approaches may be of help here. In the last chapter we set out the key strengths and weaknesses of the technical/casework and personal/partnership styles. If these suggestions are accurate, they may help schemes to identify which style has most to offer the groups they are working with. For example, if a scheme is working with people who are generally self-sufficient, but face specific difficulties or threats (asylum seekers, many users of community care services, and some users of mental health services may be examples), then a technical/casework approach is likely to be suitable. The partner can tell the advocate how they would like the issue resolved, and the advocate pursues this solution. If, on the other hand, the scheme is to work with those whose lives are substantially directed by others, or who experience ongoing disempowerment and alienation, a more personal advocacy approach may be indicated, for example citizen or certain kinds of peer advocacy.

Of course, the situation is rarely this straightforward. Personal and technical advocacy needs very often exist side by side within user groups, even within individuals. As we have suggested before, no one form of advocacy can lay claim to the full range of outcomes; schemes will need to consider whether and how they support people whose needs lie beyond the scheme's key strengths. For example, many citizen advocacy schemes, though they are geared to supporting long-term partnerships, have crisis advocates available. Similarly, a professional casework scheme might employ or liaise with a counsellor to support users who find it hard to identify choices. These efforts will be limited, though, by the scheme's need to focus on its 'core business'.

Policies, training and practice

Policies determine the boundaries of a scheme's practice. There are good examples of advocacy scheme policies to be found in *Citizen advocacy: A powerful partnership* (Wertheimer, 1998) and in *Key ideas on independent advocacy* (Advocacy 2000, 2000). These cover such elements as equal opportunities, confidentiality, and codes of practice for advocates. Schemes may also require further policies, such as health and safety and data protection, in order to comply with UK law. It is important that these policies reflect accurately the distinctive nature of a scheme. For example, a professional casework scheme which supports people with respect to sensitive and complex issues is likely to have a confidentiality policy which keeps all personal information strictly private. A citizen advocacy scheme, however, which aims to "bring the concerns of (partners) into the circles of ordinary community life" (quoted in Butler et al, 1988, p 3), may seek to strike a balance between protecting sensitive information and encouraging advocates to speak freely about their partners' interests and concerns with their family and friends.

Advocacy training is considered in detail in Chapter Seven.

Practice and credibility

Advocacy practice will be defined by all the preceding stages in the model. The scheme's management, principles and policies should all be resources from which it can draw strength when its practice is obstructed or challenged, as it almost inevitably will be. The processes outlined in the first half of the model serve not only to make advocacy happen, but to establish its credibility. Credibility is arguably an advocacy scheme's greatest resource, and one it should devote time and energy to cultivating (see Atkinson, 1999, p 35). Credibility with its user group is essential to a scheme's legitimacy; credibility with service providers is also vital, for if it is absent, advocates' arguments on behalf of partners are likely to be marginalised or rebuffed. A vital part of advocacy practice lies in establishing the 'space' in which good advocacy can happen. How do schemes present themselves to service providers in a way that promotes good communication, but is non-collusive? The information contained in *Key ideas* (Advocacy 2000, 2000, section 8) is useful in this regard, since it contains not only guidelines for the relationship between advocates and service providers (section 8.5), but also training materials to help get the message across. Nonetheless, the relationship with service providers will be defined as much by what happens in advocacy practice as by policies or agreements. There will be times when advocacy offers a real challenge to service providers, and these times may be politically difficult for the scheme involved. The fallout from these confrontations can perhaps be reduced if advocacy is also seen to reinforce and encourage good practice wherever it exists. There are many committed, skilled and empowering service workers; a balanced advocacy culture will acknowledge their contribution.

On the basis of the above, we would reiterate our argument that there is a place for the views of service providers in the evaluation of advocacy schemes, albeit a limited one. Such evaluation could establish whether service providers understand the links between a scheme's principles, practice and outcomes; for if this understanding is absent (and this may not be the fault of the scheme) the advocacy process may be limited in its scope for success.

The practice of advocacy schemes is very diverse, and the suggested model does not prescribe any one form as being better than another. A little more needs to be said here, however, about the way advocacy processes are 'owned' by the advocacy partner. We have seen that this issue of ownership highlights a key difference between technical and personal advocacy. In technical advocacy, the process is owned by the partner inasmuch as the advocate is simply an instrument for implementing the partner's wishes. Even where the advocate is informing the partner of possible ways forward, the advocate is careful to do this in an open, non-leading way. This sort of ownership can be tested by asking the partner if the advocate has followed their instructions. In personal advocacy, by contrast, it may precisely be the case that the advocate is deliberately encouraging the partner to try out new ideas and approaches, and shares in the experience of these. Of course, if the partner declines a particular idea, the advocate will respect this, but the advocate's role is not primarily directed by the partner's instructions. Rather, direction emerges from the *relationship* between advocate and partner; this empowers the partner to have greater influence in their life. As stated before, the relationship between advocate and partner is here not primarily about instruction or control but like other dynamic relationships (say with family or friends) can become the means by which a person *establishes control* over different aspects of their life.

A threat to both these kinds of practice appears where schemes (or more usually scheme funders) try to put a time limit around the duration of advocacy partnerships. This is particularly a danger, perhaps, in schemes using paid sessional workers, where the advocates' time represents a given cost outlay, but it is not unknown in volunteer advocacy schemes. To have advocates racing against time to get a 'result' is likely to compromise even the most technically-minded of schemes; there may not be time, for example, to explore all options thoroughly with the partner. It is certainly incompatible with any personal advocacy outcomes. The person-centred nature of advocacy practice needs to be defended against attempts to turn it into cheap care management.

Monitoring

The individual nature of each piece of advocacy means that it is difficult and perhaps inadvisable to monitor performance against rigid targets. If, for example, a scheme is charged with creating a number of partnerships in a year, it may be tempted to concentrate on easier pieces of work and neglect partners who are more seriously disadvantaged. Clearly, though, schemes need to be able to demonstrate to their various stakeholders that regular, useful monitoring is taking place. Though there will need to be indicators of 'outputs' (the number of partnerships or cases supported), this monitoring is likely to focus primarily on what *Key ideas* refers to as 'safeguarding quality'. Only good advocacy practice can produce good outcomes; monitoring should build as full a picture of practice as is possible, without being intrusive. Below is a list of suggested areas for monitoring:

Monitoring advocacy: areas for consideration

Outputs

Number of partnerships created/supported

Range of issues addressed by partnerships

Enquiries/identification of those needing advocacy

Waiting lists and times (where appropriate)

Quality

Partners' satisfaction with advocacy

Partners' aims

Risks to partners, advocates and staff

Vetting of new advocates

Equal opportunities

Support to advocates and partnerships

Complaints

Monitoring is not simply about collecting data: it is about interpreting it so that a picture of the scheme's current strengths and weaknesses can be established and remedial action and/or new development planned. Monitoring is therefore a lynchpin in establishing and maintaining the scheme's credibility. The issue of monitoring, perhaps more than any other, lies behind the current debate as to whether there could or should be national standards in advocacy. The potential benefit of such standards would lie in enhancing the credibility and profile of advocacy nationally, with the possibility of safeguarding key principles and achieving consistent funding. But there are objections both in principle and in practice. On the one hand, some feel that the establishment of such standards would undermine local ownership of advocacy; on the other hand, the wide range of advocacy practices calls into question whether agreement on standards could ever be achieved. The next chapter will consider these issues in more detail.

Outcomes

Chapter Three highlighted some of the difficulties that currently surround the definition and measurement of advocacy outcomes. Chapter Four suggested that it is possible to define a group of general outcomes for good advocacy. The section on 'Values' earlier in this chapter appears to confirm this conclusion; if advocacy begins with a vision, it is surely fair to ask how far a scheme succeeds in realising this vision. It may be argued that every advocacy partnership is different, and that therefore it is not possible to talk of common outcomes, but this is not so. The core values of advocacy schemes, the beliefs in equality, opportunity, justice and empowerment, derive from *shared* experiences and perceptions of inequality, disempowerment and so on. It is therefore legitimate to look for common themes in the individual results of a scheme's work; for example, in what ways is it helping people to achieve equality or empowerment?

How can schemes link what happens in individual partnerships to the more general outcomes suggested in Chapter Four? It is important to state at once that 'outcomes' in advocacy should not only refer to the 'final results' of an advocacy partnership, as would be the case if advocacy followed the service model outlined previously. 'Outcomes' refers more generally to the overall impact of advocacy partnerships, to values realised as well as to tasks done. A long-term citizen advocacy partnership for instance may have many such outcomes over the months or years of its duration.

James and Roy

Roy became James' citizen advocate a few years ago. He introduced James to his CB radio club, which James became very interested in. This shared interest really cemented the partnership. James began to tell Roy about his day centre, which he said he found boring, so Roy helped him to ask if he could try some work experience. Then James was rushed to hospital one day after collapsing. The hospital said James' hostel should provide most of his care on the ward, the hostel said it was the hospital's job. Roy helped keep the two sides talking until an agreement was reached that met James' needs.

Roy has clearly made a number of significant differences in James' life. Even with short-term partnerships, advocacy may have an effect which goes far beyond the 'issue' on which the partner initially sought help. It is important that these outcomes are identified and recorded if schemes are to show that they are not merely principled, but also effective.

How can this information be gleaned? Chapter Three discussed the potential for and limitations to gaining feedback directly from advocacy partners regarding the quality and outcomes of the advocacy they receive. User feedback will perhaps be easier to gain where the emphasis is on technical advocacy, and advocacy is the means to an agreed end. In this sort of setting, questionnaires or face-to-face interviews may help a scheme to gather valuable evidence for its impact. This approach is likely to be less effective within the context of personal advocacy, where to ask the partner to evaluate their advocate would be like asking someone to evaluate a friend. Instead, citizen advocacy schemes have developed the tradition of partnership stories, where advocate, partner and (sometimes) the scheme coordinator will reflect on the achievements of a partnership, and record them in narrative form. These stories, as was noted in Chapter Four, capture well the dramatic nature of personal advocacy, which has a human, not a service relationship at its core. But the use of anecdotes is not without difficulties in recording outcomes. First, gathering stories is a time-consuming process; it is not practicable for a scheme to tell the stories of all of its partnerships. Second, advocacy partnerships which touch on very sensitive issues are far less likely to want to tell their stories, let alone see them printed in an annual report, than those which are less difficult or intense. In (quite rightly) protecting partners from prurience and sensationalism, schemes run the risk of being left with partnership stories which seem unremarkable or anodyne. A third way for schemes to identify outcomes is for coordinators or managers to collate the information received through monitoring. At Dorset Advocacy, information about the issues addressed by advocacy partnerships is fed into a database. Every six months, a table of partnership activity is produced, similar to that suggested in the ANNETTE evaluation tool:

Measuring partnership activity

Self-esteem	22
Development of interests	28
Control of finances	21
Health/medical care	24
Training/employment	3
Accommodation issues	41
Additional paid support	6
Education needs	2
Building outside friendships	7
Negotiating with services	31
Mental Health section/rehabilitation	8
Child protection	5
Personal relationships	22
'Challenging behaviour'	30
Legal advice	10
Transport	4
Communication help	5
Changing service philosophy	5
Benefits	3
Criminal justice	4
Preventing abuse	14
Emotional support	4
Formal complaint	1
Monitoring services	2
Total	**302**

In this table, the figure beside each issue shows the number of partnerships which have actively engaged with that issue in some way during the monitoring period. The advocate may have helped the partner to identify the issue, or to bring it to the attention of service providers for the first time. They may have negotiated the issue on the partner's behalf, or have helped them to resolve or progress it in some other way. Some partnerships may have addressed only one issue during the period, other may have encountered as many as six or eight. The total figure thus gives an idea of the overall level of partnership activity.

The issues are of course not fixed, nor intended to be in any sense a standard list; they can vary from one scheme to another, and from one monitoring period to the next. This interpretation of ANNETTE allows a presentation of the full range of partnerships, and of their impact. Unlike ANNETTE in its original form, it does not bind partnerships to a narrow process of goal achievement. Some outcomes may be realised without ever having been identified as 'problems', for example where a person with limited speech starts to communicate more freely as a result of their advocate's support and attention. The table is, of course, entirely anonymous, and so avoids some of the difficulties inherent in telling partnership stories.

There are, naturally enough, difficulties with this quantitative approach, too. For one thing, it relies on the honesty of those collating the figures (although this could be verified by independent audit). For another, it gives only very limited qualitative information. Unlike feedback from partners, or partnership stories, the figures do not show the *difference* that advocacy has made to individual lives. There is no single, simple way of recording advocacy outcomes. But the three approaches described (partner feedback, partnership stories and records of issues addressed) all have something to offer. In combination, they can reveal a good deal about a scheme's impact.

How do the specific advocacy issues given in the table relate to the more general outcomes proposed in Chapter Four? This will be a matter for interpretation by individual schemes. At the most basic level, schemes might simply group individual issues under more general outcomes headings, as below:

Choice	Equality/ opportunity	Justice	Social development
Direct payments	Challenging discrimination	Supporting complaints	Changing service practices
Tailored services	Access to training		
Housing	Finding new interests	Access to law	Promoting inclusion

Support		Empowerment	Protection
Support in crises		Encouraging choice /risk taking	Preventing abuse and exploitation
Supporting rehabilitation		Promoting self-advocacy	
Help to make friends		Accessing independent living	Monitoring services

The use of the seven headings already lends a more 'qualitative' feel to the issues listed. A more sophisticated method would be to use these headings to interpret the qualitative feedback gained from partner questionnaires or partnership stories. 'Joining up' this material with informed commentary, showing how different aspects of a scheme's work coalesce around a group of core outcomes, could be very powerful.

Evaluation

The theme of 'joining up' carries over to the final aspect of the model: evaluation. If advocacy is about values in action, then values, practice and outcomes will all need to be scrutinised in a comprehensive evaluation. This is a tall order. Hitherto, advocacy evaluation systems have tended to focus on values at the expense of outcomes, or vice versa. In proposing a series of general outcomes that is as distinctive to advocacy as its principles, we are suggesting that it should be possible to map an evaluatory path from first principles to outcomes along the lines of the model suggested. If this is correct, then evaluation of advocacy schemes will not simply focus on the integrity of the different stages described in the model, but will also consider the extent to which all these stages are linked together to achieve the scheme's outcomes. The 'linking' elements in the model (ownership, policies and training, monitoring and evaluation) play a vital role in bringing principles, practice and outcomes to life.

The future development of systems for evaluating advocacy schemes will to some extent hinge on whether or not national standards are adopted by the advocacy movement. Standards could provide a series of benchmarks against which performance could be measured. This could be particularly relevant to the evaluation of scheme principles; as we have seen, there are enormous pressures to compromise within the current funding environment. If core principles such as independence, loyalty and equality were to be defined in terms of non-negotiable standards, the integrity of advocacy schemes might be considerably enhanced. But even if national standards are not adopted, the model at Figure 2 together with the seven outcomes could still provide the basis for evaluation. Here the evaluatory process could give a descriptive account of a scheme's strengths and weaknesses in turning general aims into concrete outcomes, as well as of the impact of those outcomes.

In effect, evaluation will demonstrate how far a scheme has succeeded in creating an advocacy culture within its area of operation. Has it upheld choice, and contributed to the development of a range of appropriate services? Has it effectively challenged discrimination, and enhanced the dignity of individuals? These considerations mean that it is essential that any such evaluation system should speak to audiences beyond, as well as within, the advocacy movement. Evaluation provides an opportunity to get advocacy better understood and more highly valued by interest groups, funders and society at large. The opportunity should not be squandered.

Independent evaluation is expensive. The CAIT evaluation pack, though designed to be cheaper than its predecessor CAPE, still costs upwards of £2,000 per evaluation; it is clearly not something that most schemes could afford more than once every five years or so. Though this independent input is desirable, both to check the accuracy of a scheme's claims for its performance, and to provide an objective overview, there is no reason why it should not be complemented by exercises in self-evaluation, which could reduce the workload and cost of the independent evaluators. Indeed, a complete evaluation system for schemes might include elements of external evaluation, self-evaluation, and training for schemes to help them implement the whole process correctly.

Funding

The model at Figure 2 tries to set out the parameters of an advocacy culture and to create markers by which the success of advocacy ventures may be judged. For reasons given above, funding does not appear as a heading within the model; however, it has appeared repeatedly in our discussions of the headings which do appear, just as it was a recurring theme in the previous two chapters. This is therefore a good time to review some of the ideas which have emerged in relation to the funding of advocacy, and to develop them a little further.

Service providers as funders of advocacy

It is a paradoxical but inescapable fact that advocacy is as well established as it is in the UK because of the resources it has received from service provider and service purchaser organisations; in other words, from local authorities and the NHS. Were these resources to be withdrawn tomorrow, advocacy activity in the UK would be decimated; it is highly unlikely that the National Lottery or trust sector could (or would wish to) meet more than a fraction of the shortfall. For the time being, then, the advocacy movement is likely to continue to be dependent on service organisations for its funding.

The two huge drawbacks of this situation are, as we have seen, the conflict of interest for schemes receiving money from organisations they may need to challenge, and the increasing tendency of those organisations to dictate the terms under which advocacy is to be offered, thus undermining its principles.

The Best Value culture is here to stay, and the advocacy movement must be alert to its demands. The last two chapters have tried to map out the foundations of an advocacy culture which can proclaim its own 'best value' processes. Only thus can key advocacy principles be safeguarded. There are some hopeful signs that such a culture can take root even in the present funding climate. Several local authorities have recently recruited advocacy commissioners whose task is to make sure that the funding of advocacy in their area is informed and effective, as illustrated by this recent advertisement:

Joint commissioning manager: advocacy

You will continue to shape, co-ordinate and consolidate a structured network of independent advocacy initiatives tailored to the differing specialist and cultural needs of our customers. Your role will be to lead the strategic and policy driven development of advocacy, building on the existing network of advocacy initiatives and utilising a wide range of the different forms of advocacy available. (Job advertisement, Luton Borough Council, *The Guardian*, 17 January 2001)

Even more significant in this respect is the Scottish Executive's recently published report *Independent advocacy: A guide for commissioners* (Scottish Executive, 2000). This document recognises that a simplistic approach to the funding of advocacy is inappropriate:

Traditional tendering processes are not a creative way to achieve the effective provision of advocacy. (Scottish Executive, 2000, p 23)

It recognises that different types of advocacy may be needed by different groups in different situations (pp 21-3), rather than suggesting that one model alone delivers 'Best Value'. It is to be hoped that this report will be widely read in England and Wales, as well as within its home nation.

There are two key problems with putting advocacy funding out to tender. First, unless very clear and detailed safeguards of advocacy principles are written into the specification, the tender is likely to be awarded to the organisation which does 'most' advocacy for least cost. As we saw in Chapter Three, this is likely to lead to the creation of schemes which process people, but do not effectively support them. Second, there is something a little too cosy in the idea of a local authority choosing its own watchdog; the winning scheme may feel it has to be 'tame' in order to win next year's bid. While tendering may occasionally be unavoidable, the strategic, consultative approach described in the Luton advertisement and in the Scottish 'Guide' is in general much more likely to deliver good advocacy.

Services as providers of advocacy

In the section of this chapter on scheme ownership, we noted the difficulties that can arise when advocacy is managed by organisations whose core business lies elsewhere. Although this argument was qualified, and recognition given to the skills and structural support that larger organisations can bring, it is nonetheless desirable that priority for funding be given to 'advocacy only' organisations, all other considerations being equal. This will help to reduce conflicts of interest and give a clearer definition to the concept of advocacy. A corollary to this is the suggestion that advocacy schemes should consider carefully whether it is helpful to style themselves 'services' at all. On the one hand, the term invites the assumption that advocacy can be bought, delivered and evaluated like any other community care service; this report has sought to demonstrate that it cannot. On the other hand, referring to advocacy as a service risks reducing it to the status of mere trouble-shooting, since personal advocacy – one person's commitment to another – is incompatible with the service approach. There is a real danger that the supportive, empowering and developmental aspects of advocacy will be lost here.

A long-term settlement?

Even if the more enlightened advocacy funding policies outlined above gain ground, there will be enduring conflicts and tensions in local and health authority funding of advocacy. Are there any prospects for change here? Much will depend on the success of the advocacy movement in raising its profile and credibility at a national level. The recent government White Paper for England and Wales *Valuing people* (DoH, 2001) may have a significant impact. It promises the development of a National Citizen Advocacy Network (NCAN) to strengthen advocacy infrastructure and to channel new money from central government to local advocacy schemes. If this network proves to be a credible voice for advocacy and a sustainable source of funding, it will have gone a long way to solving two of the most intractable problems besetting the advocacy movement.

However, there is still a long way to go. The funds to be channelled through the national network are relatively small, and it is clear that the government envisages a continuing and even an augmented role for local authorities as the funders of advocacy. There will be local government performance indicators showing:

> ...the amount spent by each council on advocacy expressed as the amount per head of people with learning disabilities known to the council. (DoH, 2001, p 124)

The potential for destructive conflicts of interest in the funding of advocacy will therefore persist unless either NCAN develops an expanded role and becomes the primary route for advocacy funding, or else at the very least issues clear standards to local authority funders of advocacy which will limit the potential for such conflicts in practice.

This chapter has sought to map out the foundations of a distinctive advocacy culture, and to look at some familiar debates within this new framework. In particular, it has suggested ways in which advocacy can sustain its independence, while still giving assurances on quality to the world at large. One quality issue remains outstanding: the question of national standards. It is with this question that the next chapter is concerned.

SIX

Looking at standards

In the last chapter we looked at the possibilities for developing an 'advocacy culture', and discussed some of the benefits this might bring in terms of raising the profile of advocacy, supporting good practice, and defending its core principles. This chapter will ask what role, if any, national standards should play in underpinning this culture and, if standards are desirable, who might develop them.

A standard can be defined as:

> A definite level of excellence or adequacy required. (*Chambers English Dictionary*, 1988)

There has been long-standing debate in the advocacy movement as to whether standards are relevant to advocacy. The arguments in favour of national standards can be summarised as follows:

National advocacy standards?

For	Against
Standards would define and protect key advocacy principles	National standards would undermine local ownership
Standards would strengthen the identity of the advocacy movement	Standards would drive out flexibility and innovation
Standards would promote quality assurance	Standards would undermine personal advocacy
Standards would be an aid to evaluation	

- *Standards would define and protect key advocacy principles.* A key theme of this book has been that independent advocacy is being undermined by the imposition of a service culture. National standards could help to ring-fence advocacy.
- *Standards would strengthen the identity of the advocacy movement.* At present, there are no hard and fast rules for determining what is and what is not advocacy. Standards here might prevent the term being so widely applied as to be meaningless, and could give a greater focus to advocacy networks.
- *Standards would promote quality assurance.* Adherence to quality standards may help schemes to gain users' confidence. Quality standards may also protect especially vulnerable partners, and reduce schemes' exposure to complaint or litigation. Finally, such standards may be helpful in persuading funders of a scheme's integrity.
- *Standards would be an aid to evaluation.* Having at least some uniform measures of performance could help to establish a baseline for evaluation. Though Chapter Three criticised the potentially 'competitive' implications of ANNETTE, this is not to say that *all* comparison between schemes is wrong.

The counter-arguments include the following:

- *National standards would undermine local ownership.* There is a fear that standards would lead to uniformity, with locally appropriate schemes being pushed out by a more corporate approach.
- *Standards would drive out flexibility and innovation.* The advocacy movement is still developing rapidly; 'volunteer advocacy', for instance, barely existed as a separate concept five years ago. National standards might make practice rigid and incapable of adapting to future needs.
- *Standards would undermine personal advocacy.* Having performance standards which advocates must meet, would define them as part of a 'service'; this would conflict with an advocacy that is rooted in personal loyalty, such as citizen advocacy.

Each of the arguments for and against advocacy standards is credible. Do they then cancel each other out? We would argue they do not. The preceding chapters have sought to convey the magnitude of the threats facing independent advocacy at the present time, and have argued that only positive and coherent action by the advocacy movement can alleviate these dangers. The status quo, under which the question of standards is left to hang in the air, is not an option; indeed, it is part of the problem. Just as it was suggested in Chapter Three that the absence of authoritative models for evaluation created a vacuum which is being filled by the demands of funders, so the same holds true of standards. If the advocacy movement does not generate its own standards, it is quite possible that these will be imposed, locally or nationally, as a condition of future funding.

If the advocacy movement decides *against* adopting national standards, by what other means could it defend its principles and identity? It might be argued that advocacy could survive simply as part of the wider disability rights movement. As an activity owned and defined by disabled people and other service users, it could be argued, advocacy would not need any external guidelines. Advocacy would then be just one tool in a wider campaign for equality and empowerment. Such an argument is attractive; this approach would seem at least to ensure the independence of advocacy. However, it has a major flaw. As we saw in Chapter Five, there is a vital distinction to be made between the ownership of an advocacy scheme and the control of individual advocacy processes. Creating the conditions under which individual partners, or partnerships, really control the advocacy process requires not only good scheme ownership, but also good principles and practice. In trying to define the latter, we are brought back once again to the question of standards. Though advocacy should be informed and inspired by the experiences of disabled people and by disability issues, ownership does not resolve the issue of standards.

It seems, then, that the advocacy movement may have no other option than to develop some core standards if it wishes advocacy to continue as a distinct and meaningful activity. If, as we have argued, the greatest threat to advocacy comes from pressures to compromise its principles, then it is in relation to principles that national standards would be most helpful. The main obstacles to creating such standards are:

- The difficulty in achieving agreement across the many different types of advocacy scheme.
- The need to avoid the potentially negative effects of national standards mentioned in the 'arguments against'.
- The question of which agency or agencies should be responsible for the implementation and monitoring of standards.

The third obstacle will be addressed a little later in the chapter. Taking the first two together, it is clear that if there are to be any standards which can be applied to advocacy as a whole, they will need to be few in number and tolerant of different approaches. In other words, they will be minimum standards; they will not prescribe how advocacy should be delivered, rather they will seek to define a threshold beneath which advocacy ceases to be acceptable; beneath which, indeed, it ceases to be advocacy.

How might such standards be developed?

The task of consulting across the advocacy movement would be a huge one; and, as we have suggested, there would be no guarantee of reaching a workable agreement. However, in Scotland, Advocacy 2000 did undertake just such an extensive consultation in developing the *Key ideas* pack (Advocacy 2000, 2000). In the last chapter we discussed the ways in which the six core principles, or key ideas which the pack identifies, could contribute to defining an autonomous advocacy culture. Might it be possible to write standards against all, or at least some, of these principles, so that they represent not merely a description of current good practice, but also clear boundaries for future advocacy developments?

We can try out the idea of standards by considering the first, and in many ways the most important, of the six 'Key ideas': independence. The principle is described as follows:

> Independence: There should be no conflicting interests which limit the actions of advocate and project. (Advocacy 2000, 2000, section 1, p 8)

The principle is unarguable; but it does not, by itself, say what the possible conflicts of interest are, or what constitutes a 'limitation' of an advocate's actions. Should all forms of local or health authority funding for advocacy be avoided, as the citizen advocacy program evaluation (CAPE) seems to imply? Or (at the other extreme) could a freelance advocate who is 'spot purchased' by social services to work with a service user on a fixed term basis in fact be perfectly acceptable under this principle? Without standards, the principle is hard to define – or defend.

In the box below are suggested six standards for independence

Standards for independence

1. An advocate must not be in the employment of a service received by their advocacy partner. Neither should an advocate have any other ties or loyalties to such a service.

2. An advocacy scheme may not be managed by an organisation that provides or purchases community care services within the area of the scheme's operation.

3. Representatives of local community care purchasers/providers shall not have voting rights in the management of an advocacy scheme, except during its first two years of operation.

4. Funding agreements for advocacy schemes may specify the models of advocacy to be offered, the groups to whom it may be offered, and additional general indicators of advocacy need. Funders should not stipulate or control the duration of advocacy partnerships, the means of referral, or the decision as to which individuals should or should not receive advocacy.

5. Evaluation will ideally follow an established advocacy model; where this is not the case, the terms of the evaluation should be negotiated between the scheme and its funder.

6. There should be a presumption in favour of organisations whose sole work is advocacy, or which offer only free advice, representation and informal support.

that might allow a clear and consistent understanding of the terms 'advocate' and 'advocacy scheme'.

The first of these suggested standards should be self-evident; someone who is part of a service cannot be relied on to challenge that service on behalf of another. They will have an inner conflict of loyalties, and may additionally face pressure from the service's management. Precisely the same reasoning lies behind the second standard; advocacy organisations can no more be part of a wider service system than can individual advocates, or they will experience the same conflicting pressures. There may be some debate as to what exactly constitutes a 'community care service', but on any interpretation of the term providers of local residential, day, domiciliary or healthcare services would be excluded from the provision of advocacy. The third standard seeks to strike a balance between safeguarding the independence of advocacy, and recognising that individual service workers have often played a key part in helping to launch new schemes. It is unrealistic to expect every advocacy scheme to be fully independent from day one; service representatives may be a good point of contact for management skills or funding bids. However, once a scheme is established, there are no grounds for leaving any managerial powers with such representatives; they should never, in any case, form the majority on a management committee.

The fourth standard also seeks to strike a balance between the legitimate aim of offering appropriate types of advocacy to those most in need, and the danger that such 'targeting' may become a covert means of controlling the advocacy process itself. In particular, the practice of setting a time limit to advocacy roles appears entirely incompatible with independent action on behalf of the individual. If a problem is worth taking up in the first place, it is also worth seeing through to the end – whenever the 'end' may be. This is not to say that all advocacy roles should be long term; within a casework-type scheme, issues may indeed be resolved within a short period, and the advocate's role then ends; but it is the issue which dictates the timescale, not vice versa.

The fifth standard seeks to ensure that advocacy is not evaluated according to inappropriate models which may distort both its processes and outcomes. Although advocacy evaluation systems have hitherto tended to focus on the citizen advocacy model, the new Advocacy 2000 evaluation pack aims to be applicable to a wide range of schemes, and other broadly-based systems may follow. Achieving widespread recognition and acceptance for one or more of these evaluation systems should be a high priority for the advocacy movement; only when the evaluation is seen as credible are a scheme's outcomes likely to be perceived as authentic. There may still be times, however, when no established programme of evaluation really fits a scheme's circumstances. In developing a one-off evaluation appropriate for these circumstances, it is important that the terms and criteria are agreed by both the scheme and its funder, and not simply imposed by the latter without regard for advocacy principles.

The sixth and final standard might prove the most controversial of all. The second standard does not preclude the possibility that an organisation which provides community care services in one area could provide advocacy in another (and this is, in fact, what happens with several national voluntary organisations). However, the final standard suggests a preference for structurally independent advocacy schemes, in the belief that independent advocacy is more likely to flourish in such a setting. The principle here is not absolute; in some settings the most effective advocacy may be delivered via a large organisation, but here there should be an aim to achieve structural independence for the advocacy scheme within, say, two years. The standard should not inhibit minority ethnic or campaigning groups from developing advocacy. Many groups which offer peer support to, say, disabled people or to people from minority ethnic communities find that an advocacy project complements their work in giving advice, offering support and raising public awareness. There does not seem to be any major conflict of interest here, so long as the group is not also providing care or other paid-for services.

The authors are aware that many good advocacy schemes will not currently be working to all the above standards; indeed, the authors' own schemes do not meet all of them. In particular, there may be many schemes which form part of larger voluntary organisations providing advocacy that is both credible and effective but would not meet the sixth standard. At this first stage, it needs to be stressed that the standards outlined above are not intended as a means for judging individual schemes as 'good' or 'bad'; they are intended to demonstrate a means by which the advocacy movement could 'hold the line' on the principle of independence. Were these or similar standards to be adopted (after widespread consultation), schemes may have to adapt or reorganise to meet them, but if the end result were a clearer and more sustainable definition of independent advocacy, such changes would surely be worthwhile.

Would these hypothetical standards avoid the dangers foreseen by those who argue against national standards? We believe they would. Instead of undermining local ownership of advocacy, standards 2, 3 and 6 would help to defend this by making it more difficult for providers of care to provide advocacy also. Nor would these standards limit the creativity of schemes, since they do not stipulate how advocacy should be provided. Finally, standard 4, by making the duration of the advocacy process a matter solely for the partner and scheme to agree, asserts the validity of open-ended advocacy partnerships as envisaged in the citizen advocacy model. Standards for independence, then, may have much to offer the advocacy movement.

These are only core minimum standards, intended to be applicable across all forms of advocacy. Within individual schemes, these core standards may, of course, be complemented by others relating to the particular model of advocacy followed by the scheme; this theme will be developed later in the chapter. Could similar national standards be devised for the other 'Key ideas?' One of these, 'Advocacy dilemmas' clearly could not be supported by standards, since it refers to problems which are not easily resolved, and which may not have a right answer. (Advocacy 2000, 2000, section 1, p 8).

Of the others, 'Inclusion and respect', 'Empowerment' and 'Loyalty' all have to do with the *process* of advocacy, rather than its status. They can, therefore, for the purposes of this discussion, be considered under the more general heading of the fifth principle, 'Safeguarding quality'.

The question of national *quality* standards in advocacy, even more than the question of standards for independence, is likely to raise fears about advocacy becoming a uniform, bureaucratic and soulless exercise. It is therefore worth considering some of the arguments for quality standards, to see if they stand up to scrutiny:

Quality standards would increase 'customer confidence' in advocacy schemes. This is the argument for standards which is perhaps most frequently encountered in retail and service cultures, but it is probably not that relevant to advocacy. Most people who use advocacy are hardly in a position to 'shop around' for it. What helps people put their trust in an advocate is the fact that the advocate is unambiguously on their side – not the fact that they have a Charter Mark.

Quality standards would support independent evaluation. This is true, though as we have suggested, evaluation needs to cover every aspect of a scheme's life.

Quality standards would make advocacy more attractive to funders. Though what is 'attractive' is not always what is right, it does not seem unreasonable for funders to want to be assured that the schemes they are funding will meet some basic quality thresholds. If the advocacy movement as a whole wishes to assert standards for independence, as suggested above, those who commission advocacy are likely to demand quality standards in return.

Quality standards would help to safeguard the interests of vulnerable people. If it is acknowledged that some people who receive advocacy are extremely vulnerable, then schemes have a duty at the very least to try to ensure that this vulnerability is not exploited or increased by advocacy. There is an obligation, too, to ensure that advocates are not put at unnecessary risk.

There are grounds, then, for trying to develop some quality standards for advocacy, so long as these are rooted in an overall advocacy culture and do not reflect non-advocacy agendas. Could such standards be agreed nationally so as to embrace all advocacy schemes? A major obstacle here lies in the very different ways in which the personal and technical advocacy styles are implemented. A key premise of citizen advocacy is that advocacy partnerships should be autonomous. The scheme does not direct or control partnerships; were it to do so, it would be imposing its own interests over and above those of the partner. This concern dictates the attitude to quality standards; each partnership is different, and it is up to the advocate and partner together to work out what constitutes 'good' advocacy for the partner's situation. Citizen advocacy schemes do not formally supervise advocates or review partnerships, because this would imply that the scheme was the ultimate 'owner' of the advocacy.

Technical advocacy appears more amenable to what might be termed 'service standards'. In a casework scheme, using professional advocates, advocacy is something that is provided by the scheme as a whole, usually through a system of line management. At each level of the management structure, there will be given responsibilities, for which standards might be set. For example, such a scheme might undertake to provide the first meeting with an advocate within so many days of receiving a partner's enquiry; advocates might be required to take up issues with the relevant service provider within so many days of this first meeting, and so on.

Given that this approach differs significantly from that of personal advocacy, can any common standards be developed? A useful preliminary step here may be to establish a *framework* for common standards; that is, to define the kinds of themes that minimum standards might cover. By identifying core areas of advocacy practice, we can ensure that any standards which may be developed are at least relevant, rather than merely arbitrary. Six areas suggest themselves.

Access to advocacy. It seems reasonable to require that schemes should be both *fair* in deciding who they can and cannot support, and *effective* in reaching out to a representative cross-section of their chosen client group(s). This, like all other advocacy standards, will be qualitative rather than quantitative. It should also be stated that there will never be a financial charge for advocacy.

Applying quality standards in advocacy

Access to advocacy

Advocate preparation

Advocacy processes

Coping with risk

Advocacy outcomes

Complaints

Advocate preparation. Casework schemes will generally train their advocates to a certain level of skill and knowledge, in order that they can respond competently to a range of needs. Citizen advocacy schemes tend to avoid formal training, believing that the key to effective advocacy lies in the quality of the relationship between partner and advocate. On either view, however, one can ask: what steps are taken to ensure that the advocate is suitable and competent for their role?

Advocacy processes. Here again, the differences between personal and technical advocacy are significant but not irreconcilable. Within a casework setting, there might be standards determining the speed of response to enquiries (as we have seen) or how an advocate agrees aims with the partner. Within citizen advocacy, partnerships cannot be 'standardised' in this way, but there are nonetheless boundaries for advocates' conduct, such as are set out in various codes of practice for advocates.

Coping with risk. This necessarily will involve the undertaking of risk assessments that may require the input of non-advocacy professionals with the relevant risk management experience. In all the advocacy forms, it may be tempting to play down the elements of potential risk (to both advocates and partners) in order to appear informal and 'user-friendly', but standards in this area may well help to safeguard people against bad practice.

Advocacy outcomes. Within casework schemes, standards for advocacy outcomes might imply some sort of mechanism for ensuring that the partner is satisfied with the results of the advocacy input. Within citizen advocacy, such a mechanism would not be appropriate, for here partnerships are not necessarily aimed at discrete 'results'. Rather, the partnership itself *is* the outcome, a creative and continuing source of benefit in the partner's life if it is working well. It is this 'if' that citizen advocacy schemes can and should monitor. While it may not be possible to define *standard* indicators of a good citizen advocacy partnership, there are any number of signs which can show whether a partnership is succeeding or not. Citizen advocacy schemes should have mechanisms which demonstrate that they are alert to the difference between successful and unsuccessful partnerships.

Complaints. Advocacy not infrequently involves highlighting the failures and shortcomings of care and other services. Schemes should be able to demonstrate that they, too, are open to fair challenge and constructive criticism. Anyone who feels they have been wronged by an advocate or by a scheme should have access to a complaints procedure.

So quality standards seem possible in respect of these six areas of practice, even if the precise content of the standards will vary according to the model of advocacy followed. One might go a step further, and say that this framework could be cast in the form of 'outline' standards, the detail of which individual schemes might complete, as follows:

Outline quality standards

Every scheme should record and monitor the advocacy needs of partners, in order to ensure equality and diversity of advocacy provision. (Access)

Every scheme should have mechanisms for ensuring that advocates act according to the wishes of, or out of a unique loyalty to, the advocacy partner. (Preparation/process)

Every scheme should have a written policy on confidentiality. (Process)

Every scheme should have mechanisms for identifying risks to partners, advocates and staff, and procedures for minimising these. (Risk)

Every scheme should have written procedures for meeting advocacy needs, and for monitoring how far they are being met. (Outcomes)

Every scheme should have a complaints procedure. (Complaints)

It is important to stress that these and the other standards proposed in this chapter are examples only; they are intended to demonstrate the possibility and potential value of national standards, not to dictate exactly what those standards should be. They are put forward in the belief that all forms of advocacy are interdependent, and that the advocacy culture described in the last chapter needs a degree of unity at its core, as well as a respect for diversity, if it is to flourish.

How might such national standards be implemented?

It was stated in Chapter One that no regional or national advocacy forum has hitherto acquired both the breadth of membership and the credibility needed to develop and implement such standards. But the National Citizen Advocacy Network (NCAN) envisaged in the *Valuing people* White Paper could transform this situation, and give real impetus to the development of authoritative standards, *if* it is implemented wisely.

Valuing people gives only the briefest definition of what it means by citizen advocacy, and even this is in a footnote:

> Citizen advocates (that is, volunteers) create a relationship with a person with learning disabilities, seeking to understand and to represent the person with learning disabilities' views. (DoH, 2001, p 46, note)

This emphasis on voluntary relationship is welcome. Perhaps for the first time, it signals government recognition of the validity of personal advocacy as described in Chapter Four. It is seen that some people with learning disabilities (and the same is presumably true of members of other groups) may only be able to express themselves through a partnership process that offers support, encouragement and the opportunity to develop roles other than that of 'client'.

How can this policy initiative best be turned into an effective advocacy infrastructure? In the light of what has been written earlier in this chapter, it can be argued that NCAN will need to be *both* broadly-based *and* clearly focused on advocacy principles. It will need to be broadly-based because too narrow a definition of what constitutes citizen advocacy will simply perpetuate the sectarianism that has hitherto undermined the advocacy movement. It is therefore to be hoped that *all* volunteer-based advocacy schemes will be invited to join the network, even if they do not identify with the traditional citizen advocacy model. Within this broad framework, however, principles and standards for the differing forms of volunteer-based advocacy will need to be clearly stated and maintained, in order to prevent them simply merging into an ill-considered hybrid.

That such a broadly-based yet principled approach can work has been demonstrated by the success of Advocacy 2000 in Scotland. There is no reason why NCAN should not be able to enshrine, defend and promote principles and standards for traditional citizen advocacy alongside those for what was described in Chapter One as volunteer advocacy. It is to be hoped, too, that good lines of communication can be established between NCAN and professional casework advocacy schemes; the debate about standards needs to be as broadly informed as possible.

If the national standards proposed earlier in the chapter can provide a core of unity for the advocacy movement, how might the development of standards specific to each different form of advocacy (such as NCAN may develop) impact on these different forms? To this question, the remainder of this chapter will seek to contribute some answers.

Citizen advocacy

Standards for adherence to citizen advocacy principles are, as we have seen, already articulated in CAPE, and reinforced in *Learning from citizen advocacy programs* (O'Brien, 1987) and the CAIT evaluation pack (Hanley and Davies, 1998). For many within the citizen advocacy movement, CAPE determines not only the success of a scheme, but also its validity. Only if a scheme is following, or aiming to follow, the CAPE standards, is it seen to have a right to call itself a citizen advocacy project. The standards aim to ensure that citizen advocacy is as *unlike* service processes as possible; that it admits as few as possible of those interests and procedures which allow people to be seen as anything less than people. In this sense, CAPE was the first document to set out the need for an autonomous advocacy culture.

However, as we saw in Chapter Three, CAPE has not, in fact, set the standards for more than a fraction of UK advocacy schemes, despite the citizen advocacy model having influenced and inspired many more. This may in part be because some of the standards, such as those requiring non-statutory funding, are very hard to follow in the UK. But it may also be because the very comprehensiveness of the standards appears to create a very exclusive definition of 'true' citizen advocacy. Must a scheme be fully implementing all the standards from day one in order to be a 'real' citizen advocacy scheme? Or does a smaller group of 'core' standards represent the heart of the model, so that a scheme which stood by at least these core standards could still say it practised citizen advocacy? The citizen advocacy movement has not been able to determine these questions, and this lack of agreement has probably weakened the identity of the citizen advocacy model in the UK.

The CAPE standards measure adherence to citizen advocacy principles, but not the effectiveness with which these are implemented. The wish of citizen advocacy schemes to do away with a conventional 'quality standards' approach here is understandable, given that this is rooted in a service model which they reject. However, this outlook becomes excessive if it leads schemes to banish the idea of professionalism altogether, on the grounds that citizen advocacy is 'informal'. Much of citizen advocacy is indeed informal, and this is true not just of the partnerships themselves, which often evolve as friendships, but also of advocate recruitment and preparation. Advocates are as likely to be recruited through conversations in cafes and supermarkets as they are through advertisements. Their 'orientation' may or may not include a detailed introduction to the citizen advocacy model. But citizen advocacy coordinators are not unique in this way of working. Detached youth workers or health workers may adopt highly 'informal' strategies. But this is not to say they are not professional (they may need to be more professional than most), nor that such professionalism cannot be monitored or enhanced by the appropriate mechanisms. The same is surely true of paid citizen advocacy staff.

One-sided emphasis on the 'informality' of citizen advocacy obscures the considerable professional expertise that does, in fact, exist among citizen advocacy coordinators. It could hardly be otherwise. To gain access to people deemed to be vulnerable, to listen to them, and to create the means by which advocacy can work for them requires a range of skills. It should be possible to acknowledge and reflect on these skills without undermining citizen advocacy principles.

Viewed in this light, adopting some minimum standards for coordinators' practice may convince funders and others of the considerable professional skills that exist within citizen advocacy, even though these skills are not an end in themselves but are directed to the creation of freely given advocacy partnerships. However informal their approach, citizen advocacy schemes exist for a purpose. If this is defined as matching people with disabilities and resourceful community members who would otherwise be unlikely to share their lives (O'Brien, 1987, p 15), then schemes must acknowledge an interest in, and responsibility for, the results of these introductions. If the following elements are essential to the success of partnerships, then some core standards may be possible to define them:

- selection of citizen advocates
- preparation of advocates
- agreeing the match between advocate and partner
- monitoring and supporting partnerships
- good advocate conduct.

Again, as with the uniform national standards discussed earlier in this chapter, there is a question as to which body would develop such standards, were they agreed to be desirable. Citizen Advocacy Information and Training (CAIT), the national focus of the citizen advocacy movement, has adopted the traditional approach of upholding citizen advocacy principles while avoiding any 'formalisation' of advocacy roles. The British Institute of Learning Disabilities (BILD) on the other hand has recently produced both a training pack for citizen advocates entitled *Pathways to citizen advocacy* (Brooke and Harris, 2000) and draft *Guidelines on good practice in ctizen advocacy*, both of which have a pragmatic focus on developing the *effectiveness* of advocacy. Both initiatives *could* in principle form the basis for quality standards, but both have drawn criticism. In particular, the implication that citizen advocates need prior 'training' in advocacy in general is seen as undermining the primacy of their relationship with their partner. More will be said about *Pathways to citizen advocacy* in the next chapter.

Both the principles *and* the effectiveness of citizen advocacy need safeguarding, and standards may have a part to play here – if the mechanism for developing them can be found.

Volunteer advocacy

'Volunteer advocacy' is a definition that is still taking shape. It does not refer to a precise model of advocacy, but denotes all those schemes which, while they do not support the long-term one-to-one partnerships that are at the heart of the citizen advocacy model, nonetheless see voluntary commitment as an essential ingredient in advocacy. Typically, volunteer advocates will support partners through specific issues and withdraw once these are resolved; this process may also be referred to as crisis advocacy. At its best, this approach can allow schemes to deliver some of the expertise normally associated with professional casework advocacy through a partnership which retains something of the understanding and commitment of personal advocacy.

Finding the right citizen advocate for someone can take many months; volunteer advocacy schemes are likely to have a trained advocate available at short notice. This means that volunteer advocacy can make a more immediate impact on service processes. Advocates can quickly be found to represent partners in tribunals, assessments and complaints procedures. But this strength is not without its dangers. The very responsiveness of volunteer advocacy can help to breed a 'crisis culture' in which anyone who is not in dire straits is deemed to have no need of advocacy or other forms of support. Involvement in such advocacy often yields striking results – a court case won, a benefit regained – and there will always be a need for it. Preventive or developmental approaches are less glamorous; yet it remains a fact that most people, given a choice, would prefer to avoid crises, however good the support available.

Allied to this is a danger of tokenism. Schemes are sometimes approached by services to provide an advocate 'for John's review meeting' for example. The approach may be well meant, but it carries an assumption that (a) this will be the only chance John gets to comment on his services this year and (b) that he could not possibly wish things otherwise. Advocates are for people, not for meetings, and schemes may wish to spell this out in their standards.

Areas in which volunteer advocacy schemes may wish to develop their own specific standards might be as follows:

• Who 'owns' the advocacy? Does it rest entirely with the partner and advocate, as in citizen advocacy, or is the advocate managed by the scheme? Can advocates be 'removed' from a particular piece of advocacy casework by the scheme manager? Under what circumstances?

- Who decides when a partnership should end – the partner, advocate or scheme?
- How will the scheme work with people who are less able to make their choices known?

If the scheme sees itself as 'managing' the delivery of advocacy, then standards for the training of advocates, for example, may also be appropriate. Some volunteer advocacy schemes are already exploring the possibility of external accreditation of advocates via universities and colleges, and this could yield benefits in terms of the quality and consistency of advocates' performance. Safeguards may need to be developed, though, to ensure that those who gain accreditation do not seek to pass themselves off as freelance 'qualified advocates'.

Because 'volunteer advocacy' covers such a diversity of schemes, it is hard to envisage uniform standards for them other than the sort of minimum standards which we have suggested for all advocacy schemes. However, the three areas set out above might provide a framework for standards specific to individual schemes.

Professional advocacy

As we saw in Chapter Three, Atkinson (1999) sees professional advocacy as offering a promising way forward for the advocacy movement as a whole. Government sponsorship of the Patient Advocacy Liaison Service (PALS) idea reinforces this perception; and if advocacy is made a statutory entitlement under reforms of the 1983 Mental Health Act, it is quite possible that the government will require more or less professional standards here, too. Of all the different forms of advocacy, professional advocacy appears to sit most comfortably with BestValue notions of performance, targets and outcomes. The technical advocacy approach of helping someone to get the result they want, no more, no less, seems close to conventional ideas of a service.

But is this really true? The striking thing about many professional advocates is how far they retain a 'voluntary' ethos. We know of a number of such advocates who have regularly worked way over their paid hours because of their personal commitment to the individuals they are supporting. In addition, most professional advocates will feel that their role is not simply about representing people; it is also about empowering them:

Jean

Jean is a mother who has experienced mental ill-health. She has recently been detained under the Mental Health Act, but now a discharge meeting is planned. A professional advocate, Mustafa, has acted for her throughout her detention. He asks her if she wants any help with childcare when she returns home.

"If I ask for help with the kids, they'll take them into care", says Jean.

"Social services have a duty to give you proper support", says Mustafa. "And you have every right to ask for help. I could ask on your behalf ... but it might be more effective coming from you."

Jean is not sure if she can raise the issue, but after further encouragement from Mustafa, she agrees to do so. When she makes her request at the discharge meeting, the social worker is receptive:

"What times of day are most difficult for you?" she asks Jean. Support is arranged for these times.

In this scenario, a technical advocacy problem has been solved; but just as importantly, by believing in Jean and encouraging her to speak for herself, Mustafa has helped her to begin to develop a relationship with the services that is based on need and legitimate entitlement, rather than on fear. Thus even where advocacy is supposedly at its most technical, in the professional casework setting, clear elements of personal advocacy remain. As suggested earlier in this chapter, what establishes the viability of *any* advocacy role is the fact that the advocate is uniquely 'on the side of' the person they support. Professional advocates *may* demonstrate this simply by following their clients' instructions to the letter; equally, however, they may demonstrate it through empathy or encouragement, attributes which bear the hallmarks of personal advocacy.

If this perception is correct, it confirms that however much personal and technical advocacy may differ philosophically, in practice they can never totally be separated. However tempting it may be to view casework as essentially a different form of activity from partnership advocacy, the temptation should be resisted. For if those who commission advocacy are allowed to believe that it can be neatly divided into 'problem solving' on the one hand, and 'befriending' on the other, and that they can purchase the former while dispensing with the latter, *all* forms of advocacy will be falsified. There will be a wholesale professionalisation of the concept and it will become the property of 'advocacy services' which are scarcely less remote and impersonal than the health and care services to which they were supposed to promote access. The need for coherence and unity in the advocacy movement has never been stronger; the opportunity to achieve them may not come again.

The national standards for advocacy principles suggested earlier in this chapter might help professional advocacy schemes to avoid this kind of absorption into the service culture. In particular, the standards for the independent ownership of advocacy schemes, and for control of the duration of partnerships may help to retain the essential person-centredness of advocacy. These could be supplemented by standards specific to professional advocacy. Standards covering the following areas could be useful here:

Standards in professional advocacy?

Administrative activities

The advocate–client relationship

Advocacy outcomes

Empowerment and self-esteem

Administrative activities. Is the scheme office based in an accessible location? Are there efficient and clear systems for dealing with referrals, queries and requests for information? Are waiting times kept to a minimum? Do office staff deal with enquiries in a courteous and respectful way? Are there adequate information and recording systems? Are policies and procedures clear, accessible and relevant to the work?

The advocate–client relationship. Was the advocate accessible and available at the times and places required by the client? Did they listen to and communicate with the partner in a respectful and non-judgemental manner? Did they do the things that they said they would, at the times they said? Did they honour an appropriate level of confidentiality, and respect gender and culture issues? Were the advocacy techniques appropriate to the situation? Did the client feel involved and included at all times?

Advocacy outcomes. What was the outcome of the advocacy process? Did the client achieve their initial goals? What changed as a result of the advocacy intervention? Has the client been treated fairly and equally, and been heard? Were their views acted on? Is the client satisfied with the outcome of the advocacy process? Would they use the scheme again?

Empowerment and self-esteem. Does the client feel empowered as a result of their relationship with the advocate? Are they more aware of their rights? Have they developed any sustainable self-advocacy skills? Do they feel more able to tackle problems and issues themselves in future? Have they been supported to develop their own opinions and aspirations?

Peer advocacy

Peer advocacy is still an emerging form. It centres on the belief that a shared experience of disadvantage or discrimination enables the advocate to be 'on the side' of the partner or client in a way that is particularly meaningful. Individual peer advocates may act within the models of advocacy already discussed in this chapter; that is, they may be citizen, volunteer, or professional advocates. But there are also a number of schemes devoted exclusively to developing peer advocacy where, for example, users of mental health services are supported by other users.

There is no single definition of how peer advocacy schemes should work. Not only may the peer advocate offer a partnership- or casework-based approach, the very distinction between helper and helped may be abolished in an advocacy relationship that is founded on the idea of mutual support. Hence it is not possible to suggest a single set of standards for peer advocacy. But the question of standards is still relevant. In discussing the evaluation of citizen advocacy in Chapter Three, it was suggested that a *principled* advocacy relationship is not necessarily an *effective* one. The same point applies to peer advocacy; the peer relationship may be realised and highly effective in some instances, but not so in others. There will certainly be a need for monitoring here; and individual schemes may feel that standards also have a part to play in reinforcing good practice. The United Kingdom Advocacy Network (UKAN) Code of Practice is particularly relevant, since it provides safeguards for advocacy that is wholly owned by service users.

Health advocacy

Although not a specific advocacy form, the issue of health advocacy for minority ethnic communities has gained prominence in recent years, driven primarily by a significant research project undertaken by Silvera and Kapasi on behalf of the King's Fund (Silvera and Kapasi, 2000). The research involved a mapping exercise of both specific and generic advocacy agencies that had a role in advocating for minority ethnic communities in a general health context. The authors highlighted a number of areas for action, including the development of effective networks; capacity building among advocacy 'providers'; the development and funding of policy and research in the field; improving funding and commissioning of advocacy; developing partnerships; training and awareness-raising; and the development of common standards. The last point is the most significant in the context of this chapter – Silvera and Kapasi go as far as to suggest a number of possible standards which they felt would help to raise the quality and effectiveness of health advocacy schemes:

> ... there was a clear case to develop standards that improved the organisation and delivery of services and the performance and behaviour of advocates themselves. These would provide clearer and more objective ways for assessing effectiveness. (Silvera and Kapasi, 2000, p 85)

The authors propose two sets of measures for health advocacy schemes, the first being 'essential' criteria such as customer satisfaction, basic data collection and clearly stated service aims and the second being 'added value' measures such as improved social inclusion, impact on wider service delivery and on individual health. At the time of going to press the King's Fund is now progressing to stage two of this process, by funding an initiative aimed at implementing many of the recommendations of this research.

Our discussion of advocacy standards has necessarily been both tentative and selective. Tentative, because the whole subject of standards is so contentious, and selective because a comprehensive survey of possible advocacy standards would fill a book in its own right. Nonetheless, some conclusions have emerged. First, it seems at least possible that some national minimum standards could be set for all kinds of advocacy which would not undermine scheme diversity, but which would protect some core advocacy principles, especially independence. Second, it has been suggested that different forms of advocacy, or individual schemes, could adopt further standards to support their work in general, and to combat weaknesses or imbalances in particular. In citizen advocacy, standards might help to counter an excessive emphasis on informality. In volunteer and professional advocacy, they may help to ensure that personal advocacy perspectives are at least to some extent defended, and absorption into the service culture avoided.

In relation to both volunteer and professional advocacy, the training of advocates has several times been mentioned as a quality issue. It is with differing approaches to the training of advocates that the next chapter is concerned.

SEVEN

Learning, skills and validation

So far we have focused primarily on organisational issues and processes in the development of effective advocacy. Given that the bulk of advocacy is sanctioned and supported by advocacy agencies, this is appropriate, but what about the individual advocates? At its most fundamental level, advocacy exists as a relationship between two people, the advocate and their partner. Although the advocate will have been given access to induction, training and support from the advocacy agency, they remain relatively autonomous. It is the individual advocate, not the scheme, who will be responsible for setting both the tone of and agenda for the advocacy partnership. While a key value of advocacy is that the advocate and partner work collaboratively to agree the terms of the relationship, it needs to be recognised that there exists a power imbalance between the two parties in the relationship, at least in the first instance. That is, the partner or client is in need of support or assistance, which the advocate chooses and is able to provide.

Although overly simplistic (some partners are entirely clear what they want from advocacy), this in essence is how many advocacy relationships begin. Hence the advocate carries a great duty to use their not inconsiderable power responsibly and with good intent. The role of the advocacy scheme in this context is to put in place systems to ensure that first, the advocate is aware of this responsibility and second, is equipped with the skills and insight to act in an empowering way. Different types of scheme will tend to do this in different ways.

Citizen advocacy and 'training'

There are differences of perspective and approach between citizen advocacy and other forms of advocacy whether they be volunteer or paid worker-based, in relation to training. In citizen advocacy, much greater emphasis is placed on the mutuality of the advocacy relationship, ascribing a great deal of autonomy and independence to the advocate and partner to set their own agenda and follow their own path. This is not a business transaction between a professional and a client, rather it is an equal partnership based on the key values of community and inclusion. The citizen advocate is an 'ordinary' person who brings a rich and varied life experience to the partnership and makes a commitment to utilising that experience to ensure their partner is also heard and respected as a citizen. In this sense, it is not necessary or desirable for the citizen advocate to undergo a rigorous, standardised training programme before they can be considered 'ready'. Citizen advocacy schemes place a great emphasis on the process of 'matching' advocates and partners based on common values, experiences and interests. This ensures that the advocate's unique skills and talents are put to best use, rather than requiring them to conform to a predefined set of criteria or template for what an advocate should look like.

This is not to say that citizen advocacy schemes do not offer training and support to advocates: most schemes provide induction or orientation, in part to explain the key values and principles of citizen advocacy to potential advocates but also to provide an opportunity for scheme coordinators to get to know the participants. In this way citizen advocacy schemes are able to 'select out' individuals who may not be suited to becoming citizen advocates, but who may be redirected towards some other form of voluntary work. During the course of the advocacy relationship, advocates may also be offered the chance to attend regular support groups or briefing sessions, and meet with scheme staff and other advocates to discuss issues of interest or concern.

A core belief in citizen advocacy is that marginalised people not only have a right to representation, but that this representation is most enduring and effective if it grows out of the organic and dramatic relationships which link ordinary members of the community. This is why the theme of inclusion is so fundamental in citizen advocacy: it is the foundation on which the more tangible advocacy outcomes are built. Training, by definition, seeks to 'add' something to the volunteer, be it skills or knowledge; added together, these inputs define the volunteer's role. Citizen advocacy schemes, on the other hand, feel that such 'additions' actually *diminish* the advocate's capacity to offer the partner the equal human relationship that anchors all true advocacy. Instead of committing themselves, the trained advocate is enacting a role; and the partner is yet again cheated of real human concern, and given an 'intervention' instead.

The ideals of citizen advocacy are compelling; so compelling, perhaps, that practitioners sometimes overlook the fact that they are *ideals*, and can only be achieved (or worked towards) through real, and sometimes slow, processes. So one must contrast with the citizen advocacy ideal of a freestanding, effective partnership between two citizens, rooted in ordinary human concern, the fact that many new advocates will be uncertain of their role; that they may never have negotiated with service providers before; that their partner's life may look anything but 'ordinary' at first sight. Should citizen advocacy schemes ignore these facts, and simply assume that every partnership is ideal from the moment it begins, so long as it follows citizen advocacy principles? Such a position is surely untenable. Just as it was argued in the last chapter that citizen advocacy coordinators have a level of responsibility for the quality of the partnerships they create, so it can be argued here that they have a responsibility to promote the development of advocates and advocacy partnerships towards the ideal (however that is conceived). The 'orientation' or induction of citizen advocates, and their ongoing support, may indeed need to be tailored to local, and even individual circumstances; but this is not to say that 'anything goes'.

Pathways to citizen advocacy

The *Pathways to citizen advocacy* training pack (Brooke and Harris, 2000) represents a first structured attempt at the task of developing the effectiveness of citizen advocates. It is a modular training package designed specifically for citizen advocacy schemes working with people with learning disabilities. The pack is divided into two parts. The seven 'Foundation' units in part one aim to provide:

> initial preparation and training for citizen advocates who will partner people with severe learning disabilities. (Brooke and Harris, 2000, p 2)

while the nine 'Advocacy in Context' units in part two offer:

> continued training and development of citizen advocates in ongoing advocacy partnerships. (Brooke and Harris, 2000, p 2)

The units comprise:

Foundation units

- What advocacy is about
- Disability awareness and attitudes
- Communication: getting started
- Communication: relationship building
- Choices and decision making
- Conflicts and complaints
- Approaches to problems

Advocacy in context units

- Difference and diversity
- Sexuality
- Families, friends and volunteers
- Working with professionals
- Health and learning disabilities
- Choice in where to live
- Choice in daytime opportunities
- Education and learning disabilities
- The law, learning disabilities, and citizen advocacy

Each unit is designed to last between one and three hours and includes teaching, group discussion and practical exercises such as case studies. The pack's authors recommend that, wherever possible, people with learning disabilities themselves should be engaged as trainers.

As presented, *Pathways* has a somewhat prescriptive feel. Each unit begins with a statement of 'learning outcomes':

> After completing this unit participants will be able to... (Unit F5, p 2)

Even if unintentionally, this may create the impression that citizen advocates must reach a certain level of knowledge before they are 'qualified', or that completion of the units bestows some kind of accreditation on the advocate. Either perception would undermine, not so much the principles, as the entire rationale of citizen advocacy. For here it is the match between partner and advocate, rather than any expertise the advocate holds, which is the root of the partnership.

Of course, it is important that advocates bring insight and knowledge to their partnerships, and used flexibly the modules can help advocates to reflect on, and learn about, issues relevant to their specific partners. However, there needs to be a stronger emphasis on the 'prior learning' – the ordinary life experiences – which citizen advocates bring to their role.

Again, though the emphasis on training by people with learning disabilities is welcome, the pack overall feels too much 'trainer-based'. The primary impression is very much of advocates as students and 'workers' rather than as partners and contributors. Even in the 'Advocacy in Context' units, which are designed for advocates already supporting a partner, the learning outcomes make no mention of the value of learning from partnership experiences. Again, this seems to negate the distinctiveness of citizen advocacy, which aims at empowering people through participation in community and not primarily through receipt of services. A module about encouraging advocates (and partners) to share their experiences informally and constructively might redress the balance somewhat.

Ultimately, it will be the take-up of the *Pathways to citizen advocacy* pack which determines whether or not it is successful. It is possible that, in its present form, it does not have enough of a citizen advocacy 'feel'. The pack may develop, or it may spur others to develop alternative resources for encouraging, developing and empowering citizen advocates and advocacy partnerships. At the very least, by requiring the citizen advocacy movement to focus on tasks as well as on ideals, it has opened up a large and legitimate area of debate.

Different approach, different skills?

Given that citizen advocacy is founded on the fundamental assumption that advocacy relationships are one-to-one and long-term, it is possible to be relatively confident that if the matching process is carried out well, the foundation will be laid for an effective partnership. However, in a more generic 'casework' advocacy scheme where advocates (be they volunteers or paid staff) support a number of partners, the issue is more complex. At any one time the advocacy worker may be supporting several individuals with a wide range of issues and from a variety of backgrounds. Although many such schemes have a single client-group focus (for example mental health, older people), a plethora of different experiences and problems may still arise. In this event, the 'casework' advocate needs to be both versatile and knowledgeable across a much wider spectrum. This may include housing, welfare rights, health and community care legislation and local service provision. In addition to this comprehensive knowledge of 'the system', the casework advocate also needs the full range of advocacy skills and techniques to be able to support and represent their partner effectively. This combination of skills and knowledge is seen as an essential ingredient for a successful casework advocacy approach, as shown below:

Skills	Knowledge
Active listening	Relevant legislation/rights
Empathy and openness	Local service systems
Action planning	Complaints procedures
Collaborative working	Other sources of information and advice
Negotiation skills	Key personnel
Persistence and tenacity	Range of issues and possible solutions
Communication and administration	Particular needs and wishes of partner
Evaluation and monitoring	Advocacy principles and practice

There are implications here for both the recruitment and training of advocates, volunteers or paid workers, within casework advocacy. Not only will the scheme want to consider specifying the essential skills and knowledge required at the recruitment stage, but also in relation to ongoing training and supervision. In other words, if advocates do not already possess all the requisite abilities, how can they acquire them?

Unlike traditional health and social care disciplines such as nursing or social work, advocacy does not require a specific qualification. Given that its roots are in everyday community life and social action, it is not surprising that advocacy has flourished without the need to impose rigid training programmes or minimum skills requirements. However, as the advocacy sector has grown to incorporate a much larger proportion of casework schemes using paid advocates, so the demand for more formal training programmes has increased. The impetus for training has come in part from the advocates themselves, keen as they are to provide the best possible support to users. There is also a link to quality and effectiveness, in particular the requirements of funding bodies who will often insist that advocates have access to minimum levels of training and supervision. For advocacy agencies such requirements may provide a useful tool for negotiating a reasonable level of funding for training within project budgets. There is precious little free training available to advocates, and conferences and high-level policy seminars are notoriously expensive.

Training for advocates, whether induction or ongoing, is essential for the continuous development of an individual's skills and knowledge. It also provides an opportunity to revisit core advocacy values and principles as well as offering a useful networking facility. The induction aspect of training is particularly important. It sets the context within which an advocate will operate and should, if properly coordinated, provide a grounding in both general advocacy philosophy and specific organisational practices. A typical induction programme may cover some or all of the issues outlined below:

Induction training checklist

Orientation to scheme/agency, other team members, policies and procedures, referral systems, local profile

Introduction to advocacy values and key principles

Advocacy skills – listening, negotiating, empowering

Equal opportunities and anti-discriminatory practice

Introduction to local service systems and key personnel

'Shadowing' other advocates

Administration – record-keeping, client file systems, time-keeping

There may be any number of appropriate teaching and learning methods adopted by advocacy schemes to ensure advocates have the requisite skills and attitudes. To an extent, particular agencies must have the freedom to choose from and adapt a wide range of approaches, but the advocate also has the right to expect certain basic facilities to be in place for their arrival at the scheme. Training should be an ongoing process which is not limited to an initial induction programme but which enables the advocate to learn and develop continuously. There is scope for a great deal of flexibility both in terms of the content and method of training, encompassing approaches as diverse as 'on-the-job' training, reading key texts and role play. The following is a summary of the main training methods used in a casework or volunteer advocacy context.

On-the-job learning

To a great extent advocacy skills and approaches are best learned in a real-life environment that enables both the advocate and their partner or client to contribute to and benefit from the experience. By working together to challenge a decision or resolve a dispute, both parties are in an ideal position to try out different techniques and review their effectiveness. In this way, advocates and partners gain an insight into the range of advocacy approaches (the process) and results (the outcome). The subtleties and nuances of each approach can be scrutinised and evaluated in the light of actual experiences, enabling the advocate to reflect on their practice and modify as appropriate, for example, the decision about whether to write a letter or make a telephone call to a particular professional; when and how to request a case review or reassessment; or how to articulate a particular problem the client or partner is experiencing.

This process of reflective learning can be greatly assisted by having access to a supportive manager and staff team. In such an environment, advocates are supported when making mistakes and in learning from them. In this respect, there are clear advantages to advocates being based in dedicated teams rather than dispersed in organisations for which advocacy is only one element of a range of other services. The dedicated, independent advocacy agency is well equipped to support individual advocates and develop shared learning across the team. Although it is essential that agencies have in place clear policies around confidentiality and access to information, most teams should have established systems for sharing information about particular clients in order to pool ideas and approaches.

However, there is a danger that in such situations clients can become 'guinea pigs' for the advocate's learning, especially in the case of new and inexperienced advocacy workers. Given that casework advocacy is a relatively new phenomenon this is to an extent inevitable. There is no template for effective advocacy and what works well in one situation with one person, may not work at all in another. Consider the following example:

Abdihakim

Abdihakim approaches the advocacy scheme after his attempts to get rehoused have failed. Although he believes he has a good case for a transfer to another area (he has experienced both racial harassment and verbal abuse from neighbours in relation to his mental health problems), his local housing office has failed to act and he is becoming increasingly frustrated.

Abdihakim's newly appointed advocate decides the best approach is to write to the local MP about the situation, and claims that the housing department, in not responding to claims of racial harassment, is itself operating in a racist manner. He also copies this letter to the local newspaper.

Although the approach adopted by the advocate in this example is not necessarily 'wrong', there might well be a variety of other less drastic measures that would be worth trying before going to the press. In this scenario, these may include meeting with the housing officer; arranging a case conference; seeking written support for the client's case for rehousing from social workers, GPs and others; or writing to the housing office manager.

It is not clear from this example whether the advocate was operating on the explicit instruction of the client or whether he had chosen the particular course of action under his own initiative. It would be incumbent on anyone acting in this way to ensure their client was fully informed of their rights and choices, and possible likely outcomes of any such activities. The client should always have the final say over what action is taken on their behalf, and should be encouraged wherever possible to advocate for themselves, with support.

At the heart of any concept of in-role learning should be an emphasis on learning from the advocacy partner. As stated previously, partners are the only experts in advocacy. Just as their expertise may emerge in a variety of ways, so schemes need to impart to advocates a range of techniques for learning from their partners. In some situations this will mean demonstrating to the partner that it is their views alone that inform the advocate; that the advocate will convey these views, and vigorously represent them, to whichever agency is appropriate. In other situations, the advocate may need to be much more proactive, encouraging a partner who has low expectations of life to see that better options are available to them. In suggesting these options, the advocate will need to be informed by all of their encounters with the partner, trying to see through the partner's eyes possible ways ahead. Advocates have found out their partners' interests and wishes in all manner of ways; it is important that this diversity is respected.

Role play

Another effective learning method that may have relevance to advocacy schemes is the use of role play. This involves a number of 'actors' (the training participants) adopting different roles within a given scenario and playing out those roles to their natural conclusion. Typical examples of role-play scenarios include going to a hospital appointment, and complaining about poor service in a restaurant. Each actor is briefed about their role and given cues as to how a particular character might act and react. Other participants who do not take part in the role play are asked to comment on how each person behaves in their role and what can be learned from this. At the end of the role play actors are supported to debrief and come out of role. It is also possible to replay a particular scenario with participants swapping roles in order to gain insight into what each party thinks and feels.

Role play enables advocates to experience at first hand a range of different advocacy situations and practice their skills in a safe and supportive environment. Although clearly not the same as a real-life situation, it is possible to get a sense of what it feels like to be cast in a particular role, whether that be as a service user, advocate or service provider. Role play can be a good way of conveying the energy and dynamics of advocacy although it does have its disadvantages. On the positive side, the fact that it is essentially a staged drama means that nobody will suffer if things go wrong – there are no real-world repercussions from a poorly judged advocacy intervention other than slight embarrassment and the opportunity to try again. For instance, the role-play actors may experiment with 'hard' and 'soft' approaches to particular situations such as tribunals or case conferences.

Such training might have given Abdihakim's advocate in the above story a broader sense of the options available. The advocate is able to reflect instantly on both the advocacy process and outcomes, revisit the role scenario immediately to experiment with different methods and their impact on people's behaviour, attitudes and decisions. If the role play is done in a supportive group environment, participants are also able to take feedback from other group members and observe their different approaches to the same role scenario. In this way advocates have the opportunity to compare and contrast different advocacy and representation styles.

There are some disadvantages to the role-play method of training however. It is still essentially an artificially created situation, and in real life people rarely get second chances. It also does nothing to address the key advocacy issue of relationships, in that the actors are often meeting for the first time in the role-play environment. Although a useful tool for practising representation and negotiation skills, role play does not allow for a critical analysis of the values of advocacy – it is a practice tool only. There is also the danger that, given the realistic nature of most role-play scenarios, emotions can run high and participants identify personally with their roles. For this reason, role play as a training tool requires a skilled facilitator who can support people getting into role and coming out of role. It is also essential that participants are debriefed after each session so that issues from the role play are not carried over into real life.

Classroom learning

The different advocacy forms revolve around a set of principles. These principles include such key issues as independence, autonomy, loyalty and equality, choice and the right to self-determination. It is crucial that advocacy schemes actively promote and protect these values in order that genuine, independent advocacy flourishes and survives in a constantly changing environment.

This presents a challenge to advocacy schemes – how to instil in new and inexperienced advocates a sense of ownership of and 'adherence' to these particular values. It is possible to make available to advocates the small but authoritative body of literature on the subject (see below), but this does not address the issue of shared learning and a collective consciousness around advocacy philosophy, history and practice. To achieve this, the advocacy scheme may need to resort to more traditional learning and teaching methods such as workshops, seminars and lectures, focusing on different advocacy models, principles and definitions. Other related issues which can be tackled in this way include learning about relevant legislation (such as the 1990 NHS and Community Care Act, 1989 Children's Act, and 1983 Mental Health Act), learning about local organisations and service systems, and other related disciplines such as counselling, advice, the law and mediation.

Beyond the initial induction training packages for new advocates, which are traditionally organised 'in-house' by particular advocacy agencies, there is currently a lack of good-quality advocacy training in this country. This is true both in terms of training specifically for advocates (whether citizen advocates or casework advocates) and advocacy awareness training for service providers and allied professionals. The small amount of training that is available tends to be in the form of one-day courses on particular advocacy issues such as volunteer recruitment, equal opportunities and advocating for people with particular needs or issues such as dementia. The concept of a modular, comprehensive training programme that covers all aspects of advocacy values and practice is still a relatively new one, although there are currently some pilot projects in the UK experimenting with different training packages. We have already discussed the *Pathways to citizen advocacy* pack as an example of this genre.

In East London, two different accredited training pilots are currently under way. The first is an entry-level core competency training course entitled Advocacy for Accessing Services. This course is aimed at people who have a basic understanding of advocacy issues and who want to broaden their experience. The course lasts for six weeks and on completion, students are automatically eligible for paid sessional advocacy work in the East London area. The second course, the Certificate in Advocacy, is a more advanced qualification accredited by the University of East London and covers six areas: diversity and discrimination; models and skills of advocacy; mind, body and culture; understanding socially excluded adults in society; society and health; and casework in advocacy. It is not clear whether such qualifications will have any validity in the wider advocacy field, but they provide a useful example of the direction in which the issue of accredited training is headed.

Case studies

One particularly effective learning method in classroom-based workshops is the use of case studies. These are realistic examples of possible advocacy scenarios that enable participants, often in small groups, to put into practice the theoretical understanding they have developed during the training. In this way, advocacy values are clearly linked to practice and trainees are encouraged to reflect on why and how a particular approach works. It is possible to see why, for example, advocates should avoid adopting a 'best interests' approach to representing people and instead concentrate on what their partner is actually saying they want and need. Another example would be to help trainees develop a clearer understanding of the relationship between advocacy process and outcomes, that is, the *style* of advocacy adopted may have a direct impact on the end *result*.

Reading the literature

There does exist a modest body of literature on advocacy, principally on citizen advocacy but more recently on other models such as peer or casework advocacy. Those written materials which do exist range from relatively basic introductory articles on the benefits of advocacy in a health and social care context through to detailed practical guides for anyone setting up an advocacy scheme.

A great deal of the early written work was imported from the US, primarily such influential texts as *CAPE: Standards for citizen advocacy program evaluation* (O'Brien and Wolfensberger, 1979) and *Learning from citizen advocacy programs* (O'Brien, 1987). In the UK, the first attempts to produce an interpretation of the citizen advocacy model include *Citizen advocacy: A powerful partnership* (Butler et al, 1988, revised by Wertheimer, 1998) and *Citizen advocacy: The inside view* (Simons, 1993). More recently, publications such as *Power tools* (Leader and Crosby, 1998) have provided a useful guide to local groups attempting to set up an advocacy scheme from the grassroots, and the books *Advocacy: A review* (Atkinson, 1999) and *Advocacy skills for health and social care professionals* (Bateman, 2000) have contributed to the national debate on what constitutes 'real' advocacy. There are also a number of texts focusing on evaluation of advocacy schemes, such as Advocacy Network Newcastle (1995) and the Citizen Advocacy Information and Training (CAIT) evaluation pack (Hanley and Davies, 1998).

It must be noted that publications such as those listed are often not easily accessible to individual advocates either in terms of availability or content. This is especially the case with early works on citizen advocacy as they are closely associated both by subject matter and language to the social theories of normalisation and social role valorisation. For a more detailed summary of the range of written materials currently available on the subject, refer to the References and further reading at the end of this book.

Training and accreditation

Any discussion of advocacy training should consider the question of accreditation. On the one hand, as we have seen, the government's plans for PALS and the reform of the 1983 Mental Health Act raise the spectre of a professionalised and bureaucratised version of advocacy which only those duly accredited will be able to practice. On the other, there are more positive views of accreditation emerging from within the advocacy movement. The question of standards, discussed in the last chapter, has obvious implications here; if there were national standards for advocacy, then only schemes which were accredited as meeting them would be likely to receive funding and support. More generally, the wish to develop the quality of advocacy has already led a number of schemes and educational bodies to develop locally accredited training courses.

Significant here are the courses being offered by St Andrews University in both advocacy and self-advocacy, which lead to academic qualifications. A number of advocacy schemes, too, are fostering links with local colleges with a view to developing accredited advocate training courses. Such initiatives are welcome in that they allow for the creation of in-depth courses which few organisations could match in-house. They may also provide an arena in which philosophies and experiences of advocacy could be discussed and developed, away from the pressures of day-to-day advocacy activity. But these courses raise questions, too. How is it decided what level of learning or expertise in an advocate warrants accreditation? What would accreditation mean? That the advocate can now practise within a designated scheme? That they can start their own scheme, or perhaps even begin to trade as freelance advocates, charging fees to those they 'help'? Accreditation needs more careful discussion.

There is a need for schemes to develop practical, as well as principled, identities. What advocacy is 'about' can never simply be a set of beliefs; the model proposed in Chapter Five stressed the need for the strongest possible connections between the theoretical and practical aspects of a scheme. Training clearly has a major role to play in turning principles into practice, and in refining principles in the light of that practice. It is therefore pertinent to ask:

- Would accredited training promote better advocacy?
- Should accredited training follow national norms?

There are four main benefits which might arise from accredited training:

1. *Enforcing national standards for advocacy.* If national standards of any description were to be adopted, there would need to be mechanisms for informing schemes and advocates about these. Accredited training could have a role to play in ensuring conformity with these standards.
2. *Breadth and consistency.* Accredited training could lead to volunteer and casework advocates having a broader understanding of advocacy in its different forms. Insight could be gained into key advocacy principles and outcomes which may not all be apparent within the work of their own schemes.
3. *Social and political awareness.* Accredited training would foster understanding of the wider political context within which advocacy exists, and its links to other social justice movements.
4. *Status.* Accredited training could enhance the status of advocacy and of advocates. Nationally endorsed courses might provide good opportunities for networking and the sharing of good practice.

Each of these arguments carries some weight. However, the benefits envisaged in 2 and 3 do not necessarily *depend* on the existence of accredited training, and would certainly not require national uniformity. As regards 1, the national standards suggested in Chapter Six were more related to advocacy principles than to advocate performance, so training is not a key issue here. Finally, 4 may well set alarm bells ringing! If the advocacy movement allows concern with the status of advocates to usurp its concern for the status of partners, a very questionable kind of professionalism creeps in; surely the last thing that advocacy partners need is the creation of a Royal College of Advocates.

The main difficulty with an uncritical move towards accreditation is that it is likely to lead to confusion between *preparation for*, and *legitimisation of* the advocate's role. It is entirely proper that volunteer and casework advocacy schemes should wish to maximise their advocates' effectiveness by developing their learning and skills; but such training does not 'make' an advocate. In a sense, advocacy only really exists in the situation where one person stands by another, either with the latter's consent, or else in single-minded commitment to their interests. The relationship between personal and technical advocacy is significant here; however much advocacy is described in terms of skill, awareness, and technique (and each of these is important) there is an irreducible personal element in all genuine advocacy which cannot be codified or explained away. It is this personal element – this consent, this commitment, this trust – which gives advocacy its legitimacy.

If training only prepares advocates for their role, but does not legitimise that role (in the way that, say, a teaching certificate permits someone to teach) the case for standardised national training for advocates is further weakened. Preparation of advocates will need to have regard to local circumstances as well as the wider picture. In any case, the gulf that exists between the citizen advocacy standpoint on training, and that of volunteer or casework schemes, makes any unified system for accrediting advocates impossible. With citizen advocacy, as we have seen, accrediting individual advocates would subvert the form, although accreditation of *schemes* remains a possibility.

Does this mean that the accreditation of casework and volunteer advocates is a dead end? Not at all. As was suggested earlier in this chapter, creating links between advocacy schemes and academic environments could be a source of insight and renewal. The development of high-quality training should be welcomed, and it seems only right that the completion of such training should be recognised in some way. But training is not a panacea; it may contribute to quality in advocacy, but it does not guarantee it. There is no single set of skills, no single set of answers, which will spare advocates and advocacy schemes the need to be constantly alert to the shifting cross-currents of personal and technical advocacy.

The difference between the citizen advocacy and volunteer or casework advocacy approaches to training has been a recurring theme of this chapter. At first sight, the difference could scarcely have been more marked: on the citizen advocacy side, a refusal to train advocates on principle, on the other side an enthusiasm for any inputs which might lead to more effective advocacy. As the chapter has progressed, the difference has endured, but it has become narrower. On the one hand, it was argued that citizen advocacy schemes do have a responsibility to develop skills and resources which will help advocates and partnerships to develop, indeed that such development is essential if citizen advocacy ideals are to be realised. *Pathways to citizen advocacy* marked a first, not entirely satisfactory attempt to support such development. On the other hand, it was argued that some of the more ambitious hopes for training and accreditation for volunteer and casework advocacy need to be tempered in the light of the distinction to be drawn between preparing and authorising advocates. This distinction was related to a key theme of previous chapters: that there is at the heart of all forms of advocacy a gap that is only filled by the trust, or consent, that is established, when one person stands by another.

EIGHT

Conclusion

Writing a book about advocacy was never going to be easy. Writing a book about advocacy that attempts to move forward the debate within the advocacy movement has been harder still. Advocacy as a concept is at best open to interpretation and variation, at worst prone to corruption, dilution and ultimately, rejection. Despite the many and varied attempts of both UK and US proponents of advocacy, there remains an ambiguity about what advocacy actually is, what it achieves and how it should be done. Some forms of advocacy (such as citizen advocacy) are relatively well developed, with a clearly stated philosophy, guidelines for practice and mechanisms for review and evaluation. Others, like peer advocacy, exist only as pragmatic, informal approaches that define who the advocates are rather than what they do or how they do it.

The same discrepancies occur in the structure and organisation of advocacy. There is no standard model of an advocacy agency that is accepted across the board – rather, there are as many variations as there are local schemes. Some advocacy agencies are set up as completely autonomous and independent bodies, with multiple sources of funding, local management and high levels of user involvement. Others exist as departments within large service provider organisations funded under contract by the local or health authority. Others still occupy the middle ground between these two extremes. Although many within the advocacy movement would aspire towards the former model and are actively working towards it, the reality is that much of what currently happens in the name of advocacy is far from the ideal of complete independence and freedom from conflict of interest.

That is not to say that the efforts of individual advocates are constrained to the point of being ineffective. As we have demonstrated in previous chapters, there is more to independence than structural separation from provider agencies. Advocates (and their partners) must feel empowered to *act* autonomously whatever the circumstances, if necessary in spite of the structures and procedures that surround them. This takes us back to the fundamental basis of advocacy – the relationship between two people, the advocate and partner, and an unshakeable emphasis on dignity, respect and justice. The methods may vary but the aim should be constant.

This work has sought to describe in detail the current dilemmas and challenges facing the advocacy movement in the UK. These dilemmas are primarily ones of methodology and of organisation, although they also incorporate the specific and contemporary preoccupation with standards and regulation. But what are standards if not a tool for measurement, and what is regulation if not a process of enforcement of these measures? Advocacy is a publicly funded activity and as such warrants monitoring and evaluation. Is the money being spent in the most effective way possible? Do users get what they want from advocacy? In fact, do users even *know* what they want or what their options are? It is a challenge for those of us developing advocacy to ensure that we have the means to answer these and other questions both in terms of how advocacy is organised and also how it is implemented.

There follows a summary of the key issues raised in each of the preceding chapters in an easily accessible format. The summaries comprise a description of the current situation; an analysis of the main issues and problems; a number of recommendations for future consideration; and a series of questions which remain unanswered (and hence could form the basis for subsequent work). How this work is taken forward is for those individuals and groups within the advocacy movement to decide. But take it forward we must, for advocacy is too important to be left in the hands of those that do not care about it, are not *passionate* about it.

The significance of advocacy

The current situation

There is a wide range of advocacy schemes in the UK. Not only do these schemes support different groups of people, they work in very different ways. In some, all advocacy is undertaken by volunteers; in others, the advocates are professional caseworkers. Some advocacy partnerships support the partner for as long as they wish; in other instances, advocacy is provided just to help people sort out particular problems.

Problems and difficulties

There is no single, simple answer to the question 'What is advocacy for?' This creates a danger of misunderstanding between different forms of advocacy. The many different messages as to what advocacy is really about are likely to confuse the public, policy makers and potential funders, and this may lead to advocacy being marginalised or distorted. Chapter Four suggested that there are two contrasting, and sometimes conflicting, approaches at work in advocacy: the personal and the technical. Personal advocacy is rooted in one person's natural capacity for identification with another; technical advocacy is based on an agreement that the advocate will pursue the partner's wishes. Though different schemes will tend to emphasise one or other approach, they are nonetheless interdependent.

Recommendations

There is a range of advocacy outcomes which includes:

Choice	Access
Justice	Social development
Support	Empowerment
Protection	

- Different forms of advocacy may offer the right way for some groups to achieve these outcomes, but may be less relevant to others.
- Having different types of advocacy available within a given area is likely to be a sign of strength, not weakness.
- There is a danger that funders may only see the need for technical advocacy. The advocacy movement needs to address this danger.
- Schemes need to identify a range of means by which they can record advocacy outcomes.

> ### Topics for discussion
>
> - Does your scheme lay greater emphasis on personal or technical advocacy?
> - Which of the outcomes are achieved within your scheme? How are these outcomes identified and recorded?
> - How does the work of your scheme relate to what other local schemes are doing?

An advocacy culture: towards a distinctive identity

The current situation

There are a number of different forms of advocacy, and many different types of organisation providing advocacy. Some are independent schemes that provide only advocacy, others may be part of local 'umbrella' organisations such as Councils for Voluntary Service (CVS), or of regional or national agencies, some of which also provide care services. Advocacy is substantially funded by local authorities and the NHS; it could not be wholly funded by the trust sector.

The local nature of most advocacy schemes makes it difficult to organise national or regional initiatives to develop advocacy.

Problems and difficulties

Funding from statutory agencies presents two major problems: conflict of interests and loss of independence.

It is difficult for advocacy schemes to challenge the organisations that fund them. They may therefore not be effective in representing partners in these situations. With such funding is likely to come a requirement that advocacy is managed, delivered and monitored in line with other forms of service provision. This may undermine the independence of advocacy, and the loyalty of advocates to partners.

The advocacy movement struggles with these threats because it has no clear identity of its own. There is a need to define, not only principles, but all the processes which contribute to good advocacy.

Recommendations

- The outline model in Chapter Five could be used as a theoretical framework for defining advocacy and for developing advocacy schemes.
- A preference should be established for the provision of advocacy through 'advocacy only' organisations.
- A consensual approach to advocacy funding should be adopted where possible, and competitive tendering be used only as a last resort.
- Advocacy schemes should consider whether, in referring to themselves as 'services', they are sending misleading signals to their partners and their funders.

Topics for discussion

- Is advocacy distinct from service provision?
- Is the model suggested in Chapter Five relevant to your scheme? Does it apply to other schemes?
- How could examples of good practice in the commissioning and delivery of advocacy be collected, so as to inform regional and national policy making?

Evaluation: measuring the impact of advocacy

The current situation

There is a small number of designated advocacy evaluation systems. These tend either to focus on a scheme's adherence to advocacy principles, or to have a narrow focus on 'results'. Some schemes have independent evaluations carried out by consultants. Many schemes have never been evaluated, and rely on routine monitoring to demonstrate their worth. Formal evaluations tend to be expensive.

Problems and difficulties

Statutory funders of advocacy schemes are increasingly demanding evidence of Best Value. Since there is no agreed definition of what constitutes good advocacy, there is a danger that too much emphasis will be placed on simplistic measurement of 'throughput' and 'results'. This may lead to entirely invalid comparisons between different forms of advocacy. Worse still, it may lead to the rationing of advocacy, with schemes only allowed to support partners for a few weeks at most. This would destroy the principle of advocate–partner loyalty.

Recommendations

- The advocacy movement should develop its own models for monitoring and evaluation.
- Different models of evaluation may be appropriate for different forms of advocacy.
- New types of evaluation could be based on the outline model described in Chapter Five. Evaluation should cover *all* aspects of a scheme's work.
- Evaluation should be transparent and credible. Evaluation systems need to be promoted so that they are recognised and accepted by funders and other interested parties.
- Evaluation should not be too costly.

Topics for discussion

- How can new systems of advocacy evaluation be created, or existing ones developed?
- What is the best way to establish the credibility of a system for advocacy evaluation?
  - consensus within the advocacy movement?
  - funding from a research body to develop and pilot the system?
  - government backing for research and development?
  - devising a marketing strategy?
- What sort of evaluation would be right for your scheme?

Training

The current situation

Advocacy training tends to be organised on a scheme-by-scheme basis and is linked to the particular form of advocacy. In citizen advocacy, training is usually provided by scheme coordinators by way of orientation for potential citizen advocates, who may also be given opportunities to engage in further training if they so wish. Training for professional casework advocates may include sessions on advocacy and negotiation skills, relevant legislation and local service systems. Training takes many forms including traditional classroom learning, reading, role play and 'on-the-job' training.

There is no nationally accredited training programme for advocates, but new training initiatives are beginning to appear. BILD's *Pathways to citizen advocacy* is one example. Elsewhere, universities are starting to develop both academic and practical courses, sometimes in partnership with local schemes.

Problems and difficulties

There is some concern within the advocacy movement that accredited training would be the first step towards the 'professionalisation' of advocacy. Within citizen advocacy schemes, the concept of 'advocate training' is anathema in that citizen advocates are ordinary people who bring their own skills, knowledge and experiences to the advocacy relationship. Many citizen advocacy schemes do not even use the term 'training' to describe the support offered to advocates, preferring 'orientation'. Although many casework advocacy schemes place great emphasis on training, it is not in the traditional sense of professional career development. Rather, training equips advocates with the knowledge and skills necessary to provide effective advocacy support to a wide range of advocacy partners. There is no consensus on what this training should consist of or how it should be provided. This may be appropriate given the local nature of the majority of advocacy schemes, but has the disadvantage of being ad hoc and not necessarily well designed or delivered. Hence, not only do advocates receive training which is inconsistent, but also advocacy partners have little idea what to expect from their advocate.

There are two further issues that warrant consideration. First, it is a fact that there are now many hundreds of paid advocacy workers in the UK, and those workers, if they are to be retained within the advocacy sector, will require incentives of which training may be one element. Second, statutory funders of advocacy schemes may well see accredited training as a benchmark of quality and effectiveness and therefore insist that schemes sign up to comprehensive advocacy training programmes as they emerge.

Recommendations

Many of the existing advocacy networks mentioned previously in this book have training as a high priority. As a result, it is highly likely that we will see a proliferation of pilot accredited training programmes over the next couple of years. This is no bad thing; pilot schemes provide the opportunity to learn from mistakes and build on successes. However, there is a danger of duplication and a corresponding waste of precious resources if those pilots are not linked up in some strategic way.

It is not clear whether any of the existing national networks is in a position to take a lead on the issue of training – but without leadership, mistakes, overlap and duplication are inevitable. It is essential that the advocacy movement appoints a national lead agency for the coordination and dissemination of advocacy training pilot schemes. It would also be advantageous to map both the existing pilots and also potential funding sources and partner agencies for the delivery of accredited training at a national level.

It is important that citizen advocacy schemes are not penalised for their principled stance on training. Funders need to understand why citizen advocacy adopts such a stance and should value the role played by citizen advocates in the lives of devalued people. The advocacy movement as a whole should be prepared to defend citizen advocacy and ensure that a 'two-tier' system of advocacy is not allowed to develop.

Advocacy standards

The current situation

There is no consensus about whether national standards would strengthen or undermine the UK advocacy movement. It is possible to list both advantages and disadvantages of a system of national advocacy standards. However, the advocacy movement faces many threats to its identity and standards may present one way of demonstrating both internal coherence and external effectiveness. If the movement itself does not initiate standards they may well be imposed by funders working to a Best Value agenda. Different forms of advocacy may require different approaches in terms of the mechanisms used to define quality and effectiveness.

Problems and difficulties

There is a danger that national standards would undermine local ownership of advocacy schemes. There is also the issue of who is best placed to lead the debate on standard setting, given that none of the existing national advocacy bodies has such a mandate. It is difficult to envisage a set of standards for advocacy which has relevance to all the different advocacy forms.

Recommendations

- The advocacy movement, and in particular the new National Citizen Advocacy Network, should take the lead on developing a set of standards for advocacy which are both robust and acceptable.
- These standards should cover:
  - access to advocacy
  - advocate preparation
  - advocacy processes
  - coping with risk
  - advocacy outcomes
  - complaints
  and above all should define the concept of independence.

- There should be a working group established which includes representatives from all the existing advocacy networks to take these issues forward.
- Standards should be developed which reflect and are relevant to the different advocacy forms.

Topics for discussion

- How do we involve advocacy partners and service users in the debate about standards in a meaningful way?
- Is it possible to devise standards that both meet funders' requirements and are appropriate to advocacy schemes?
- What if advocacy schemes do not meet the pre-agreed standards?
- What infrastructure support exists to help schemes improve their practice?

Agencies designed to support people who face difficulty or disadvantage work under considerable pressures. Not the least of these is a shortage of resources. The political currents of the past 20 years have consistently flowed towards lower taxation, and in doing so have substantially eroded the belief in the comprehensive provision of free health and social care. It is hard to think of a government initiative on the NHS or community care in that time in which the intention to save money, or at least to spend it more 'efficiently', has not been a prominent feature. New regulations, too, and the need to adopt new interventions and working practices, have left many of these agencies highly managed and specialised.

There are some excellent services available; and few would wish to return to the segregated and institutionalised care arrangements that characterised the welfare state of the mid-20th century. However, these services are more obviously rationed than ever before. Access to housing, benefits and hospital surgery is rigorously scrutinised. Services strive not only to meet needs, but also to manage them, and in this they have a conflict of interests. It is the task of advocacy to bear eloquent witness to this conflict, and to the toll it exacts on people's lives. The district council which refuses permanent accommodation to a homeless single parent may be gatekeeping its service admirably, and yet be committing a real injustice. It may be cheaper for a local authority to place a disabled person in a hostel rather than support them at home; but what price that person's citizenship?

The more an individual is dependent on the support delivered by agencies working under pressure, the less they are likely to ask for. Their situation conveys to them the unspoken message 'be grateful for what you have'. Where needs are managed and not met, low expectations prevail. Personal advocacy, which is most visible perhaps in citizen and peer advocacy, challenges this climate by offering the partner relationships and opportunities outside of the service–client ethos, through which the partner can regain self-confidence and articulate higher expectations. Technical advocacy promotes the partner's wishes by outflanking or demolishing the rules, arguments or structures placed in their way.

Criticism is implicit in advocacy. If it is to highlight the many instances where people's needs are managed but not met, if it is to speak up for those who would otherwise be ignored, it cannot be part of the routine structures of care provision. Independence is for this reason the hallmark of true advocacy, for independence creates the space in which criticism can be formulated. This work has tried to show what independence means in advocacy, and how it may best be maintained and enhanced.

To say that advocacy is critical is not to say that it is negative, or worse still self-righteous. Criticism can mean endorsement as well as challenge. It refers above all to a process of testing; in the case of advocacy, testing services and attitudes against the needs and wishes of the individual. The critical nature of advocacy means that it will always be developing, and will always be diverse. Different situations highlight different advocacy needs, and diversity can be a sign of vitality. However, if advocacy is to be something more that a series of well-meaning aspirations, it must also be self-critical. Just as advocacy schemes have found a range of ways in which one person can take the side of another, so they must identify ways in which to record, reflect on, and improve these 'results'. Only in this way can advocacy lay claim to the public resources it will need in order to flourish.

Ultimately, however, the significance of advocacy relates to much broader questions than those pertaining to national standards or any specific measurement of its impact. At the heart of advocacy is a respect for the dignity of the human person, and a belief that voicing this respect can have a transforming effect on both the individual and on society at large. Advocacy is a living reminder of the possibilities of democracy where this is understood, not as majority rule, but as the accountability of all social structures to that which is best, and most profound, in the human person.

References and further reading

Advocacy 2000 (2000) *Key ideas on independent advocacy*, Edinburgh: Advocacy 2000.

ANN (Advocacy Network Newcastle) (1995) *Introducing ANNETTE*, Newcastle upon Tyne: Newcastle Council for Voluntary Service.

Atkinson, D. (1999) *Advocacy: A review*, Brighton: Pavilion.

Bateman, N. (2000) *Advocacy skills for health and social care professionals*, London: Jessica Kingsley.

Bebbington, E., Feeney, S, J., Flannigan, C.B., Glover, G.R., Lewis, S.W. and Wing, J.K. (1994) 'Inner London collaborative audit of admissions in two health districts: ethnicity and the use of the Mental Health Act', *British Journal of Psychiatry*, vol 165, pp 743-9.

Brandon, D. with Brandon, A. and T. (1995) *Advocacy: Power to people with disabilities*, Birmingham: Venture Press.

Brooke, J. and Harris, J. (2000) *Pathways to citizen advocacy Parts 1 and 2*, Kidderminster: BILD Publications.

Butler, K., Carr, S. and Sullivan, F. (1988) *Citizen advocacy: A powerful partnership*, London: National Citizen Advocacy.

Campbell, P. (1991) 'Mental health self-advocacy in the UK', in V. Franson (ed) *Mental health services in the United States and England: Struggling for change*, London: MIND Publications.

Chappell, A.L. (1992) 'Towards a sociological critique of the normalisation principle', *Disability, Handicap and Society*, vol 7, no 1, pp 35-51.

Conlan, E. (1994) *Advocacy Code of Practice*, Sheffield: UKAN.

DETR (Department of the Environment, Transport and the Regions) (1999) *DETR Circular 10/99: Local Government Act 1999: Part I Best Value*, London: DETR.

DoH (Department of Health) (2000) *The NHS Plan: A plan for investment, a plan for reform*, London: DoH.

DoH (2001) *Valuing people: A new strategy for learning disability for the 21st century*, London: DoH.

Fernando, S. (1991) *Mental health, race and culture*, London: Macmillan.

Francis, E., David, J., Johnson, N. and Sashidaran, S.P. (1989) 'Black people and psychiatry in the UK', *Psychiatric Bulletin*, vol 13, pp 482-5.

GLAD (Greater London Association of the Disabled) (1995) *The GLAD guide to advocacy*, London: GLAD.

Hadlow, J. (1996) 'Citizen advocacy observed: tool or tokenism?', *Journal of Community and Applied Psychology*, vol 6, pp 403-8.

Hanley, B. and Davies, S. (1998) *CAIT: Citizen advocacy evaluation pack*, London: CAIT.

Klijnsma, M.P. (1993) 'Patient advocacy in the Netherlands', *Psychiatric Bulletin*, vol 17, pp 230-1.

Leader, A. and Crosby, J. (1998) *Power tools: A resource pack for those committed to the development of mental health advocacy into the millennium*, Brighton: Pavilion Publishing.

MIND (1992) *The MIND guide to advocacy in mental health: Empowerment in action*, London: MIND Publications.

O'Brien, J. (1987) *Learning from citizen advocacy programs*, Atlanta: GA: Georgia Advocacy Office.

O'Brien, J. and Wolfensberger, W. (1979) *CAPE: Standards for citizen advocacy program evaluation*, Toronto, Canada: NIMR.

Read, J. and Wall Craft, J. (1994) *A guide to advocacy for mental health workers*, London: MIND/UNISON.

Robson, G. (1987) 'Nagging: models of advocacy', in I. Barker and E. Peck (eds) *Power in strange places*, London: Good Practice in Mental Health.

Rogers, A. and Pilgrim, D. (1996) *Mental health policy in Britain: A critical introduction*, Basingstoke: Macmillan.

Sang, B. and O'Brien, J. (1984) *Advocacy: The UK and American experience*, London: King's Fund.

Scottish Executive (2000) *Independent advocacy: A guide for commissioners*, Edinburgh: Scottish Executive.

Silvera, M. and Kapasi, R. (2000) *Health advocacy for minority ethnic Londoners*, London: King's Fund.

Simons, K. (1993) *Citizen advocacy: The inside view*, Bristol: Norah Fry Research Institute, University of Bristol.

UKAN (United Kingdom Advocacy Network) (1997) *Advocacy: A Code of Practice*, London: NHS Executive.

Ward, L. (ed) (1998) *Innovations in advocacy and empowerment for people with intellectual disabilities*, Chorley: Lisiev & Hall.

Webb, B. and Holly, L. (1992) *Citizen advocacy in practice*, London: Tavistock Institute.

Webb, B. and Holly, L. (1994) *Evaluating a citizen advocacy scheme*, Findings, Social Care Research 52, York: Joseph Rowntree Foundation.

Wertheimer, A. (1996) *Speaking out: Advocacy and older people*, London: Centre for Policy on Ageing.

Wertheiner, A. (1998) *Citizen advocacy: A powerful partnership*, London: CAIT.

Williams, P. (ed) (1998) *Standing by me: Stories of citizen advocacy*, London: CAIT.

Wills, A. (trans) (1956) *The notebooks of Simone Weil*, London: Routledge.

Wolfensberger, W. and Zahira, H. (eds) (1973) *Citizen advocacy and protective services for the impaired and handicapped*, Toronto: NIMR.

Index